SNACK BETTER, FEEL BETTER

Healthy snacks for remote and isolated workers

Leigh-ann Onnis

This book contains nutritional information but does not replace personal health advice offered by a medical or health professional.

ISBN: 9798665081977

Cover design by: Leigh-ann and Rob Onnis
Cover photography: Rob Onnis

Printed in the United States of America

CONTENTS

PREFACE

When I first conceptualised this book in 2019, my aim was to develop a flexible guide for healthier eating for people who live and work in geographical remote locations. Research suggests that the further people live from a capital city the poorer their health outcomes, and diet is an important factor in health outcomes. So I wanted to write a book to take the hard work out of it for those who would love some ideas about easy ways to eat healthy within the scope of life as a worker in remote areas across the globe!

From my experience working with people who live and work in remote and isolated areas of northern Australia, I knew that accessing fresh food in a regular or routine way is not always easy. Therefore, my aim was to develop a range of healthy snack ideas to suit the needs of the individual person, in way that made it easy to track how well your food choices were providing you the range of nutrients needed for a healthy body and mind.

I started by creating a list of the key criteria to ensure that the book best meets the needs of someone who is in a remote or isolated area.
   a) Ideally snacks need to be non-perishable.
   b) Some snacks can have options to add fresh fruit and vegetables (if available)
   c) Suggest combinations so that the essential nutrients can be consumed over a five-day period.

d) Ensure that there are snacks for a variety of diet preferences, including vegan, vegetarian and pescatarian diets (vegetarian diet with fish and shellfish)

In developing the criteria, I wanted to acknowledge the challenges experienced by workers in remote and isolated areas. I wanted to highlight that I understood that even with the best of intentions it can be difficult to make healthy choices where the availability of ingredients is limited. My intention was to write this book and then to develop a range of resources to make it easier for people who work in geographical remote areas.

Then... 2020 happened. As I sit and write this section of the book, I am only allowed to leave my house for essential activities, such as grocery shopping and medical appointments. In other countries, people are facing total lockdowns and have spent weeks confined to their homes. A trip to the supermarket is not an option for them at this time. All of a sudden, this is no longer an idea, it is our current reality. While I still have access to fresh foods, it is not unrealistic to imagine a time where we may need enough non-perishable nutritious food to sustain us and maintain good health while in isolation.

The audience is now broader, and the need is more pressing; yet, the original intent remains relevant. If you would like an easy guide to nutritious healthy snack options, comprised mainly of non-perishable ingredients read on...

INTRODUCTION

'Life doesn't move in straight lines, and neither does a good conversation.'

Margaret Wheatley

The best way to use this book is to think of it as a conversation with a friend. A good friend, one that offers some good advice when you ask for it, not one of those friends who believes that they are an expert on what you should be eating. In writing this book, I am drawing on my training as a naturopath, which is based on the philosophy that we are all individuals, and any changes we choose to make need to have holistic benefits. Any changes we make need to be good for our mind, body, and spirit. What do I mean when I say mind, body, and spirit? I mean that the choices you make about what you eat each day need to make you feel good about yourself (mind), they need to provide the nutrients you need to function (body), and they need to nourish you, your sense of you, so that you can be the best version of you (spirit) ... Start by considering food as medicine, what you eat can make you feel worse or better. I hope that you choose better.

We have different family histories, we all live our own lives in our own ways which leads to different health concerns ... and different relationships with foods. If you are working in rural, remote and isolated areas, and are aware of the difficulties in accessing fresh fruit and vegetables and the limited choice of foods in local shops, keep reading. If you have a busy working life and find yourself reaching for the 3pm sugar rush to get you through the day, keep reading. If you are self-isolating or quarantined in your home with the shelves relatively empty in the few shops that are still open, keep reading. If you want to eat foods that contain the essential nutrients for life, but don't want to put much time or effort into it, this book has been written for you!

This book is divided into four sections. We start with an introduction to the essential nutrients and the essentials for healthy snacking, including tips for preparation, storage and gadgets that help remote workers to make healthier snack choices. I am assuming that most people just want to get to the snacks, but I know that there are some people who would like to know more. So, in Section One, there is a summary to give you a brief description of the essential nutrients, and in Section Three each nutrient is listed with more information, including some of the best sources of each nutrient for people who work in remote and isolated areas. Section Two is where you will find the snacks, separated into categories, each with an overview of the nutrient content. Finally, Section Four contains resources and planners to help you to track how well you are including the range of essential nutrients in your snack choices.

SECTION ONE: THE NUTRIENTS

'I regret eating healthy food today – said no-one ever'

Anonymous

CHAPTER ONE: LET'S GET STARTED

<u>Introducing the essential nutrients</u>

To maintain a healthy weight, people need to balance the amount of energy they consume through food and drink with the amount of energy they use each day. Calories are a measure of how much energy is contained in the food or drink. An ideal daily intake of calories varies depending on age, metabolism and levels of physical activity, and several other factors including: gender, lifestyle, body composition (weight and height), hormones, medicines and some illnesses.

To find out your nutrient or energy requirements, a calculator is available on the Australian and New Zealand Governments' Nutrient Reference Values website, https://www.nrv.gov.au/nutrients-energy-calc. Further information is also available on the Eat for Health website, https://www.eatforhealth.gov.au/eat-health-calculators. The average energy intake varies between individuals, so use the calculator as a guide. Please see a healthcare professional for personalised advice.

Generally, the recommended daily calorie intake is approximately 2,000 calories a day for women and 2,500 for men.

The majority of the energy consumed from food comes from the macronutrients: proteins, carbohydrates and fats. These nutrients deliver energy in varying amounts. Fat is the most concentrated source of energy (9 calories per gram), followed by protein (4 calories) per gram), and carbohydrate (4 calories per gram) (FAO 2004). The energy used component of the equation describes the amount of calories the body uses to 'stay alive' (e.g. digestion, breathing, etc) and for activity.

Recommended daily nutrient intake

There are several ways to describe the recommended amount of nutrients that people need to consume each day to maintain a healthy body. In this book, I have used the Recommended Dietary Intake (RDI) which is the level of intake of essential nutrients required to sufficiently meet the needs of most of the healthy population (approximately 98%), according to age and gender (NHMRC and MOH, 2017). For some nutrients I have used Adequate Intake (AI) which is the recommended daily nutrient intake when the RDI cannot be established (due to a lack of available scientific evidence) (NHMRC and MOH, 2017). In general, AI is the same as RDI, but less reliable because the science is not yet in.

This book has been written for working people so the snacks have been developed for adults of working age (range 19-70 years). For those outside this range the snacks will still be relevant; however, the calculations for how well they meet the RDI or AI will need to be adjusted. Younger people require more nutrients at particular stages of growth, and for some nutrients, there will be different requirements for pregnant and lactating women, and for people aged over 70 years. Hence, while the proportions presented in this book have been calculated as accurately as possible, they do not supersede advice from a medical or health professional specific to your individual health needs.

Vitamins and Minerals

Vitamins are classified as being either 'fat-soluble' or 'water-soluble' which describes how the vitamin is absorbed and removed from the body. Fat-soluble vitamins are soluble in lipids (fats) and oils, and travel through the lymphatic system

Vitamins are either fat-soluble or water-soluble.

of the small intestines and circulate within the body in our blood. The fat soluble vitamins (vitamins A, D, E and K) are stored in body tissues. Water-soluble vitamins (B vitamins (folate, thiamine, riboflavin, niacin, pantothenic acid, biotin, vitamin B6 and vitamin B12) and vitamin C) dissolve in water, and therefore, cannot be stored by the body. Because they cannot stored, the body cannot store excess amounts of water-soluble vitamins for later use in the way that fat-soluble vitamins are stored. Therefore, daily intake of water soluble vitamins is important for good health.

Essential vitamins
The 13 essential vitamins needed to maintain good health are:
- Vitamin A (Retinoids and Carotene)
- B Group Vitamins - Vitamin B1 (Thiamin), Vitamin B2 (Riboflavin), Vitamin B3 (Niacin), Vitamin B5 (Panthothenic Acid), Vitamin B6, Vitamin B7 (Biotin), Vitamin B9 (Folate), and Vitamin B12 (Cobalamin)
- Vitamin C (Ascorbic Acid)
- Vitamin D
- Vitamin E
- Vitamin K

Essential minerals
There are twenty-one essential minerals, which are divided into two groups – five essential major minerals, and sixteen trace minerals. The five major essential minerals for good health must be included in the diet because they are required for healthy bodily functioning. They cannot be produced by the body. Therefore, it is important that they are provided through the foods that you eat.

The five major (or macro) essential minerals are:
- Calcium
- Phosphorus
- Potassium
- Sodium
- Magnesium

Trace minerals

The trace (or micro) minerals are essential; however, the human body only needs them in much smaller amounts. The essential trace minerals are: arsenic, boron, chloride, chromium, cobalt, copper, iodine, iron, manganese, molybdenum, nickel, selenium, silicon, sulfur, vanadium, and zinc

In this book, the trace, mineral 'iron' has been included in the nutrient table for two reasons. Firstly, the body uses iron to transport oxygen to your lungs and muscles, which not only supports overall health, for remote workers it helps you to be able to physically do all that you need to do! Also, women of child bearing age often do not get enough iron in their diet, so it is good to be aware of the amount of iron being consumed daily so that food choices can be adapted (if needed).

Non-essential minerals

There are a few minerals that are believed by some (but not all) to be needed for good health; however, at this point in time the evidence is not sufficient for them to be considered essential minerals. The non-essential minerals are: lithium, aluminum, fluoride, nickel, antimony, rubidium, cadmium, and stannum.

Nutrient Tables

This book is based on a naturopathic philosophy where the diet should include whole foods and limit processed foods. When the diet is rich in whole foods, the fats are more likely to be unsaturated, and the carbohydrates from fruits come with fibre unlike carbohydrates from junk foods like chips and chocolate.

A nutrient table is included with the snacks to show the nutrients contained in that snack. Where the snack contains foods that could vary in size or type (e.g. bananas, carrots), the nutrient table will only show the presence of the nutrient. Where the snack is made using a recipe described in this book, the approximately proportion of the RDI/AI for an example gender/age group for each nutrient will be listed in the nutrient table, together with a list of the nutrients in the snack that meet less than one percent of the prescribed RDI/AI. The age groups 30-50 years and older than 50 years were used in this book.

The quantity of each nutrient will differ between individual food items, and brands for packaged products. The quantity that used will also create a variance in regard to the proportion of the RDI or AI; however, it is unlikely that the presence of the nutrient will change (unless specifically stated for a particular snack).

	ESSENTIAL VITAMINS													ESSENTIAL MINERALS (and Iron)					
	A (RETINOL)	B1 (THIAMIN)	B2 (RIBOFLAVIN)	B3 (NIACIN)	Vitamin B5	Vitamin B6	B 7 (BIOTIN)	B9 (FOLATE)	Vitamin B12	Vitamin C	Vitamin D	Vitamin E	Vitamin K	CALCIUM	MAGNESIUM	PHOSPHORUS	POTASSIUM	SODIUM	IRON

This book contains generalised information, so the tables in this book should only be used to guide your snack choices.

The nutrient table provides a snapshot of the nutrients for each snack. In Section Three, there is a summary (customised for remote workers) of all of the nutrients, including good sources of each nutrient, and the recommended dietary allowance for the nutrients to meet the needs for an average person. In addition, you will find daily and weekly planners to track your snacks to help improve your daily consumption of a range of nutrients.

<u>Nuts, seeds and healthy fats</u>

Many of the recipes in chapters four, five and six contain nuts and seeds. Overall, nuts and seeds increase the energy content of snacks which may concern anyone who counts calories. However, nuts and seeds contain healthy fats (mostly monounsaturated and polyunsaturated fats). Research suggests that the human body does not fully digest all of the healthy fats found in nuts (it is es- 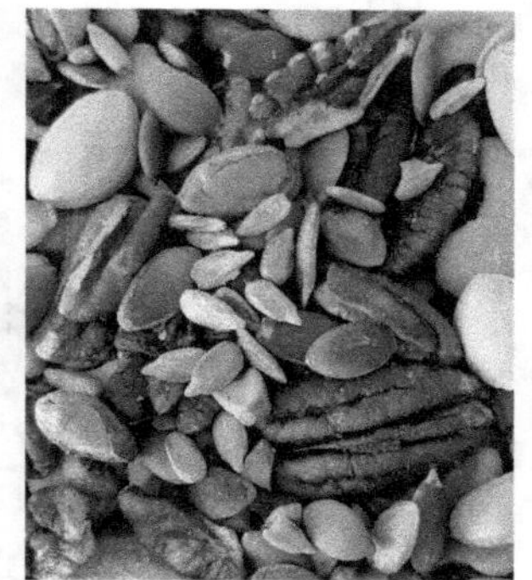 timated that approximately 68-94% are absorbed) making the fat content less concerning than the saturated fats found in animal-based foods. Nuts are high in dietary fibre, contain phytochemicals that act as antioxidants, and are rich in vitamins such as vitamin E, B-vitamins (B6, niacin, folate) and minerals such as magnesium, zinc, calcium, copper, selenium, phosphorus and potassium. Similarly, most seeds have high levels of protein, healthy fats, dietary fibre, B-vitamins (B1, B2, B3), vitamin E and minerals such as magnesium, potassium, calcium, and zinc.

Further, regularly eating nuts and seeds has other known health benefits, including: helping to maintain a healthy weight, and reducing the risks for heart disease and diabetes.

The recipes in this book use nut and vegetable fats (e.g. coconut oil) as far as possible so that the recipes are suitable for a variety of diet choices (e.g. vegan); however, some recipes do contain dairy products (e.g. butter, milk). Where dairy products are listed, please substitute with the alternative suggested (e.g. replace regular butter with cocoa butter) if you prefer a dairy-free or vegan snack.

CHAPTER TWO: PREPARATION AND EQUIPMENT

'By failing to prepare, you are preparing to fail.'
Benjamin Franklin

In writing this book, it is assumed that the reader is interested in a healthier diet, one rich in vitamins and minerals. Therefore, it is assumed that you are willing to make some effort towards preparing healthy options; however, I realise that you are busy working people so you may not always have time for food preparation. Therefore, this chapter contains ideas for everyone - from dehydrating your own fruit and vegetables to purchasing ready-to-go food items. My guess is that most people will settle for something somewhere between home-made and store-bought.

Preparing ingredients at home
Let's get started with the healthiest, purist options available. These will suit those who want to start from scratch so they know what is going into their snacks, and is good for those who prefer to avoid preservatives, artificial flavours and hidden chemicals.

Food dehydrators
If you have access to electricity and have a home-base (or somewhere you can store equipment), a food dehydrator might be a good investment. Food de-

> It is still possible to eat healthy snacks even if you are far away from fresh fruit and vegetables.

hydrators are a great way to dehydrate fruit and vegetables to add to trail mixes, soups, balls, bites and bars. All you need to do is you chop fruit and vegetables into slices and then leave them on the trays to dehydrate. The end result is dried fruit and vegetables that do not need to be refrigerated so you can take them out on the road with you or add them to other snacks (e.g. soups, trail mix).

While food dehydrators range in price, the ones at the cheaper end can do the job of dehydrating for one person quite well. If you are not sure, an investment of AU$30-40 should do the job well enough for you to decide if dehydrating food is for you!

Oven-dried
Another option is to make oven dried fruit and vegetables but these often retain some moisture and may not last as long without refrigeration. If you were travelling, you could always take a small air tight well sealed container of oven-dried produce in olive oil with you.

Preserving
Fruits and vegetables can be preserved for future use by preserving them when they are fresh. Most people will be familiar with images of rows of jars of preserved produce on shelves, which is the ideal way to do your preserving, but these storage solutions can be adapted for those travelling, particularly where it is not ideal to take glass on outback corrugated roads, or through windy mountain ranges. If you have a home-base it is best to store securely in mason jars. Then, use one jar at a time, portioning the contents into smaller snack containers.

Battery-operated kitchen appliances
If you like the idea of breakfast on the go, you might find a battery operated blender, whisk or milk frother useful. These appliances are a great way to make smoothies, or mix breakfast drinks on-the-go.

Containers and packaging

Vacuum Sealers
Vacuum sealers suck the air from a specially designed plastic bag, thus, extending the life of the contents. These are a great way to store portions so that they are ready to go. Vacuum sealed containers are another option for travelling. The special seal in the lid allows you to add a gadget and remove the air from inside the container using a hand pump (no electricity required).

Small stackable or collapsible containers
Small containers or compartmentalised containers are a great way to keep individual ingredients separate until you want to combine them. It is also a good way to measure quantities in advance. If you choose small individual containers try to get ones that stack inside each other, or collapsible containers. This will save room when packing your bag for the day (or the trip).

Reusable storage bags
Reusable storage bags are good if you don't have to worry about ingredients being squashed (e.g. nuts) and some can double as a bowl or plate at snack time.

Insulated drink containers
An insulated drink container is good for smoothies. They will keep your breakfast drinks colder for longer. This will minimize the risk of microbial activity in the drink container, and it will taste a whole lot better cold!

Utensils
Consider investing in a bamboo cutlery set, it is more robust than plastic, and can usually be carried in your hand luggage.

SECTION TWO: THE SNACKS

'Our food should be our medicine, and our medicine should be our food'

Hippocrates

CHAPTER THREE: NO FRIDGE, NO WORRIES

Not everyone has time for cooking and food preparation each week, so it is important to have nutrient-rich, easily accessible options available too. This section contains pre-packaged snacks available from most stores that do not need refrigeration. The nutritional value of these packaged foods will differ between brands; however, they will also be a better nutritional option than typical roadhouse snacks – soft drinks, flavoured milk, fried foods, and flavoured crisps/chips.

Pre-packaged packs of snacks

Fruit and vegetable chips

Many fruits are available in dried chips that are healthier options to regular high calorie, low-nutrient chips. They are available as pre-packaged snacks in supermarkets and other similar food shops. The most popular varieties are banana, apple, beetroot, sweet potato, and mango.

Fruit, vegetables and dip

Many fruits and vegetables do not require a refrigerator during the day (e.g. carrots, snow peas, apples, bananas) so they can be used as 'dippers'. If you choose a dip such as nut butter which does not need to be refrigerated and you can take this healthy snack with you to work. If you have a compartmentalised container you can keep cut carrot sticks with the nut butter neatly in one container. If you choose whole fruits, put the nut butter in a small container, and cut the whole fruit when you are ready to eat it.

Nut butter could be spread along one side of a banana adding protein to your snack and making the snack more interesting than plain fruit.

Dried fruit
Fresh fruit is always best, but it can be hard to cut and store fruit when you are on the road or frequently moving around as part of your work. In these cases, you can still gain most of the nutritional benefits by packing dried fruit instead. Please buy unsweetened, packaged dried fruits to avoid excess sugar consumption.

Fruit squeeze packs
Fruit in a squeezable pouch may look like something you would give your toddler but these handy packs can help adults to get a daily dose of fruit when access to fresh fruit is limited. Choose prepackaged fruit made with 100% real fruit, and avoid added sugars and too many chemical additives. Check the pack (or the manufacturer's website) for the nutrient values.

Smoked jerky
Dried meats, such as beef jerky, are a good way to get some additional protein in your diet and having a long shelf life they are a great snack for remote workers. Choose your brand wisely and be careful as they can contain a lot of sodium.

Protein Bars, Muesli Bars, and Health Bars
Choose high protein, low carbohydrate bars where possible. Dairy-free and vegan options are also available in most large supermarkets and health food shops. Pre-packaged protein bars are delicious and are marketed as nutritious, but be careful because they can be high in sugars, sodium and other chemical preservatives. These products may not be widely available in some rural and remote areas, but their portability makes them easy to transport (unless they are chocolate covered and you work in a warm climate).

Bliss balls
If you do not have enough hours in a day to make your own protein balls, don't worry there are many nutritious pre-packaged options available. Some are called bliss balls, others are called protein balls, regardless of the name they can be a versatile nutritious healthy treat. They are usually filled with energy-boosting ingredients, such as dates and nuts, they are definitely a healthier option than chocolate bars for those people who crave something sweet in the afternoons. Most do not contain any processed sugar so they are a good source of energy to get you through the day.

Seeds
Seeds are easy to store, do not need refrigeration and are easy to eat on the move and most seeds are an excellent source of protein. They can be combined with other foods for trail mixes, and can be added to balls, bars and bites if you are going to make your own snacks.

Air-Popped Popcorn
While popcorn is not the most nutritious food to eat alone, it is travel friendly because it is very light. It will add some fibre, and is low in calories if it is air-popped (try to keep away from the high calorie buttered varieties). Adding flavours like a sprinkle of cinnamon for a sweet treat, or a sprinkle of turmeric, chilli flakes, or Moroccan spice for a savory snack will add nutrients to the snack without adding a lot of calories to your day.

Crackers and Rice Cakes
Not all crackers are equal, but some can provide a nutritious snack, especially if paired with a nutrient dense topping (e.g. nut butter, canned tuna, sun-dried tomatoes). Look for high fibre, low calorie crackers. Puffed rice based crackers can sometimes be a good alternative to wheat-based crackers. Rice cakes can also make a great base for a snack, or can be eaten by themselves for a less tasty but satisfying snack.

Trail Mixes
Pre-packaged trail mixes are an easy way to add more nuts and seeds to your diet. These are usually great sources of protein; however, check the package carefully to avoid high sugar flavourings. Also, remember to watch the amount that you are eating because it is easy to consume a lot of trail mix without knowing if you are grazing throughout the day.

Tuna Pouches, Tinned Tuna and Tinned Salmon
There are many brands of individually packaged flavoured tuna pouches and canned fish filled with protein, omega-3 fatty acids and other nutrients depending on the flavour. Canned fish is packaged in spring water, brine or oil. Tuna and Salmon in spring water is lower in calories. If you prefer canned fish packed in oil, products using olive oil are the better option.

Fruit Leather
Fruit leather is non-perishable dried snack packed with fibre. Fruit leather can be high in sugars, so check the pack and be careful not to eat too much at once. Fruit leather is a better snack option than fried potato chips, but it is not up there with the healthiest of snack foods.

Squeeze snack packs
This product is great for people on the move who would like a wet snack. Some are high in fibre, and if they contain superfoods, such as chia seeds, they may be high in other essential nutrients too. Make sure that you check the sugar content and try to keep away from high calorie squeeze packs. A good choice I notice in my local supermarket contained chia seeds, and was rich in fibre, omega-3, calcium, and iron (70 calories).

Whole Fruit
Whole fruits are the ultimate prepackaged nutrient dense food. So if you have access to whole fruit that would last for a day with-

out refrigeration (e.g. apples, pears) or fruit that does not require refrigeration (e.g. bananas, oranges) these should be eaten regularly.

Water is #1
It is important to consume enough water each day to remain hydrated (essential when you work in hotter climates). Water is also a great way to reduce snack consumption - sometimes quenching your thirst can reduce your desire for a snack! You can add nutrients to your water with a squeeze of lemon or lime, or pop in some cucumber or mint and let the flavour infuse. These are subtle low-calorie ways to add to flavour to water. If you choose pre-mixed flavours or juices, make sure you check the sugar content.

Herbal Teas
Herbal teas are another great way to stay healthy. There are a variety of herbal teas, many of which have been reported to have therapeutic benefits. Some herbal teas, such as Japanese green tea are a great source of antioxidants. Many herbal teas are also great as iced teas, such as lemon and ginger which is superb on ice!

Made with love by You
Pre-packaged options are convenient, and sometimes more cost effective if you would like a small quantity or would like to try something new without too much time commitment. For many busy people they are the preferred snack; however, for others, they are the last resort when circumstances limit access to fresh ingredients and home cooking. This section contains snacks that need a little bit of time and effort to combine them, mix them, make them or bake them. The recipes all fall into the 'easy to make' category, and have been simplified as much as possible. Several contain substitutes so that you can switch out items according to your taste and accessibility of the items. Where the items can be frozen or stored, the snacks could last a few weeks.

This is a great option if you fly in and out from a home base, or if you are living in a remote community because most of the raw ingredients are non-perishable so they won't spoil while being transported.

How to add more nutrients into the snacks that you make

When making snacks at home, it is possible to add extra nutrients into the healthy foods you are making. Nutrient dense ingredients include:

- Psyllium husks can be added for more dietary fibre
- LSA (Linseeds, Sunflower seeds and Almonds) which is a course powder high in dietary fibre, protein, healthy fats (including omega-3) and vitamin E.
- Protein powder can be added to many recipes and is often a good replacement for cocoa
- Spirulina usually comes in a powder derived from seaweed. It is a nutrient dense food that can be added to smoothies and drinks (and is relatively tasteless).
- Maca Powder (also known as Peruvian Ginseng) is nutrient dense and can help to improve energy levels.

Trail mix

Trail mix was originally created as a portable snack for bush walking or hiking but you don't need to be on a trek to reap the benefits of a nutritious trail mix combination of fruits, nuts, seeds, grains, spices and if are not counting calories, you can even add some treats! The best part about trail mix is that it can be mixed to your preferred taste. In chapter nine, there is a table with a summary of the anticipated nutritional benefits of some of the suggested ingredients. These are provided as a guide because there are differences between brands. Also, every individual nut, grain and piece of fruit will have a different exact value of each nutrient.

There are no rules which sounds like fun, but it means that some combinations can pack a hefty calorie punch, especially if you are prone to mindlessly munching on snacks at work. If this sounds like you, it is recommended that you pre-pack your serving sizes, and never spend the afternoon alone with the entire container of trail mix!

Some of the key ingredients
While everyone's tastes differ, there are some key ingredients worth highlighting, including a few tips for those new to making Trail Mixes.
- Honey: Lightly coat the nuts and lay them on baking paper to dry before adding to the mix.
- Nuts: Try to choose unsalted, unsweetened nuts to keep sugar and sodium intake lower.
- Seeds: If you prefer not to eat nuts, seeds contain many of the nutrients found in nuts.
- Dried fruit: Be careful because the sugar content can add up quickly. Look for dried fruits low in added sugar with few preservatives.
- Grains: Choose whole grains where possible and try to avoid highly processed cereals because they add unnecessary sugar and sodium.
- Treats: Sometimes we all need a little something sweet. If choosing chocolate, 70-85% dark chocolate is a good choice and it will add extra antioxidants too.
- Extras: Adding spices is a great way to add flavor. Season your mix with sea salt, curry, ground ginger, cinnamon, nutmeg, cardamom, or cayenne pepper.

How to build a healthy trail mix
1) Select ingredients
2) Put the ingredients in a large bowl and mix well.
3) Store in an air tight container where it will keep for approximately one month.
4) You can either take the amount you require each day (e.g. one cup) or prepackage the mix into small snap lock bags (e.g. 5 x 100g per bag)

Basic Trail mix
100g almonds
100g macadamias
100g pumpkin seeds
100g pitted dates (chopped into large chunks)
100g banana chips
½ tsp cinnamon

The Basic Trail Mix Table shows the estimated proportion of the RDI/AI for each nutrient where there is 1% or more of the nutrient contained in the trail mix. These percentages are based on the daily requirements for an average 30-year-old male and female; and an average 50-year-old male and female. In Section Three there is information and templates to show how these proportions were estimated.

There are approximately 540 calories per 100g Basic Trail Mix: 11.5g Protein; 32.7g Carbohydrate; 42.3g Fat; and 7.7g Dietary Fibre. The following table shows the percentage of RDI/AI in 100g of Basic Trail Mix (%).

Gender and Age Group	Essential Vitamins											Essential Minerals (and Iron)				
	A	B1	B2	B3	B5	B6	B7	B9	C	E	K	CALC	MAG	PHOS	POT	IRON
Male >30/>50 years	7	27	22	11	9	14/11	4	5	4	54	2	11	40/38	18	17	34
Female >30/>50 years	9	29	25	12	14	14/12	4	5	4	77	2	11	51/50	18	23	15/34

The Basic Trail Mix contains approximately 1% of the AI for sodium (based on the lowest daily AI) and less than 1% of the RDI/AI for vitamins B12 (0%) and D (0%) for both males and females for the selected age groups.

The TM1 summary table shows that a 100g portion has 11.5g of protein which is 7% of the RDI for males and 9% of the RDI for females. Eating protein is a good way of feeling full for longer which is handy on those long road trips, and when it is a long time between breaks.

While this is not a low-calorie health snack, it is a better choice than some of the alternatives.

Tip: It is easier to portion the snacks if the ingredients add up to 500g

For example, 100g of a popular brand of plain potato chips (crisps) contains 559 calories with only 4.5g of protein, and few other nutrients.

Cherry Tree Trail Mix
100g roasted almonds
100g unsalted cashews
75g sunflower seeds
75g pumpkin seeds
50g unsweetened, unsulfured cherries
100g chopped **82%** dark chocolate (remove for dairy free option)
¼ tsp sea salt
½ tsp cinnamon
¼ tsp nutmeg

There are approximately 560 calories per 100g of Cherry Tree Trail Mix: 16.2g Protein; 24.1g Carbohydrate; 45.1g Fat; and 4.7g Dietary Fibre.

The following table shows the percentage of RDI/AI in 100g of the Cherry Tree Trail Mix (%)

Gender and Age Group	Essential Vitamins											Essential Minerals (and Iron)					
	A	B1	B2	B3	B5	B6	B9	B12	C	E	K	CALC	MAG	PHOS	POT	SOD*	IRON
Male >30/>50 years	4	29	24	15	9	23/17	13	3	3	105	13	11	63/60	40	18	22	74
Female >30/>50 years	5	31	29	18	14	23/20	13	3	3	149	15	11	81/78	40	24	22	33/74

*based on lowest daily AI

The Cherry Tree Trail Mix contains less than 1% of the RDI/AI for vitamins B7(0%) and D(0%) for both males and females for the selected age groups.

ACDC Trail Mix

100g roasted almonds

100g unsalted cashews

50g chopped pitted dates

20g chopped 70-85% dark chocolate

There are approximately 482 calories per 90g of ACDC Trail Mix: 14g Protein; 34g Carbohydrate; 34g Fat; and 7g Dietary Fibre. The following table shows the percentage of RDI/AI in 90g of the ACDC Trail Mix (%).

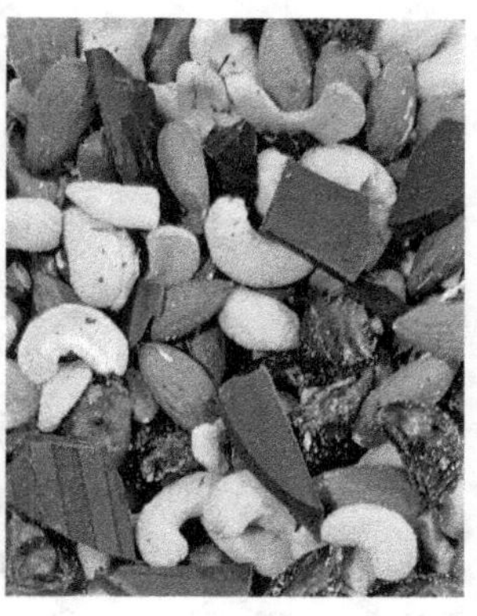

Gender and Age Group	Essential Vitamins									Essential Minerals (and Iron)				
	A	B1	B2	B3	B5	B6	B9	E	K	CALC	MAG	PHOS	POT	IRON
Male >30/>50 years	3	18	30	12	10	15/12	7	90	18	12	53/50	39	16	55
Female >30/>50 years	4	20	36	13	16	15/13	7	129	21	12	68	3	22	25/55

The ACDC Trail Mix contains approximately 1% of the AI for sodium (based on the lowest daily AI) and less than 1% of the RDI/AI for vitamins B7(0%), B12, C and D(0%) for both males and females for the selected age groups.

The summary tables show that all three trail mix combinations contain a third (or more) of the RDI/AI for Vitamin B2, and the minerals - phosphorus, magnesium, and iron. Also, 100g of each of the three trail mixes contains 100% of the daily AI for vitamin E. Summary tables have been provided to show the difference between the mixes. If you would like to roughly calculate the nutrients for you Trail Mix combinations you can use the Tables in Section Four using the nutrient estimates in the table 'An overview of the nutrients contained in individual Trail Mix ingredients'. Alternatively, use the nutrition panel on the packets of nuts and seeds and the template in Section Four.

To get you started, here are some more suggestions for other Trail Mix combinations.

Make it Over the Mountain Mix
For more energy, combine goji berries, sea salt, pistachios, dried blueberries, flaxseeds, and dark chocolate.

Tropical Northern Trail Mix
Feel transported to a vacation get away with each bite of this trail mix combination of macadamia, coconut flakes, dried mango, and cacao nibs.

Mango Madness Trail Mix
For a taste of paradise, whip up a mix of cashews, Brazil nuts, dried mango, coconut flakes, and banana chips.

Beyond the Beach Trail Mix
If you can't take a trip right now, bring the vacation to you. Combine macadamia nuts, white chocolate chips, dried pineapple, dates and coconut flakes.

Colder Climate Trail Mix
Keep the buzz going with hazelnuts, almonds, raisins, and dark chocolate-covered coffee beans.

Ocean Indulgence Trail Mix
For wholesome mix with a touch of sweetness, mix almonds, dried cherries, dark chocolate chips, sea salt, and cinnamon.

Rainforest Trails
Capture the tropical rainforest climate, with a mix of banana chips, peanuts, almonds, dark chocolate chips, raisins, and coconut flakes.

CHAPTER FOUR: HEAT REQUIRED

The squares, balls, bars and bites in the next few chapters make great snacks for people on the go, and people who don't have access to shops, kitchens or other sources of fresh fruit and vegetables during the day. The snacks have been chosen because of their high protein content which helps to reduce your appetite, and supports many important bodily functions, including metabolism. Where fresh fruit and vegetables are available, it is suggested that whole fruits be chosen as snacks to compliment the benefits of high protein snacks. Fresh fruit and vegetables that may be available in remote areas and travel well in day packs include: bananas, apples, pears, oranges, grapes, blueberries, kiwi fruit and carrots.

Hot-plate needed to melt or mix

The snacks in this section have ingredients that need to be melted. An electric stove-top is ideal; however, a camping stove would do the job if you are camping or in a remote location. Some need refrigeration as well.

Chocky Nutty Roadblock Bites

The best way to describe these is high protein chocolate crackle! Add puffed rice for the full experience.

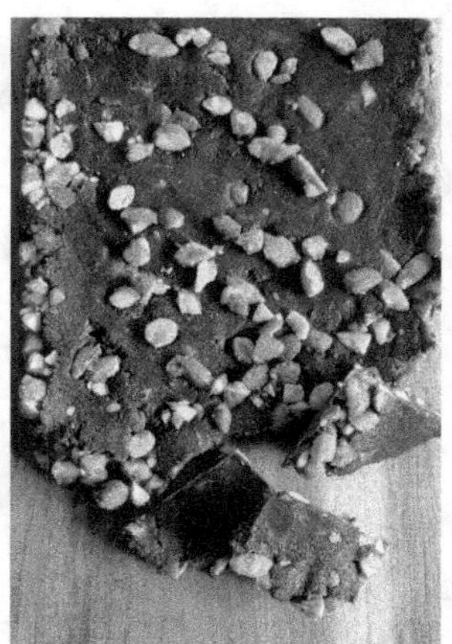

What you need:
2 tbsp water
200g unsalted roasted almonds
¼ tsp sea salt
20g butter (can be substituted)
100g cocoa butter
50g unsweetened cooking chocolate
200g powdered Artificial Sweetener (e.g. Natvia in Australia, Swerve in USA)
2 scoops (approx 80g) chocolate protein powder
½ tsp vanilla extract

How to make it:
1) Roughly chop the almonds and sift the Artificial Sweetener.
2) Combine 100g of the artificial sweetener, and water in a saucepan and stir gently until the mixture boils.
3) Continue to cook until the mixture darkens. The mixture will smoke slightly; so keep your eye on it.
4) Remove mixture from the heat. Add the 20g butter and 160g almonds, and stir quickly making sure the almonds are coated by the mixture. Stir in the sea salt.
5) Spread the almonds out onto baking sheet
6) Melt the cocoa butter and chocolate in a saucepan on a low heat until it is smooth.
7) Add the other 100g of sifted Artificial Sweetener and chocolate protein powder and stir until combined.
8) Remove chocolate mixture from heat and stir in the vanilla extract.
9) Mix with the almonds and spread the mix onto baking paper.
10) Sprinkle the remaining 40g almonds and some sea salt (optional) over the top and put into the fridge to set.

11) When the mixture is hard (approximately 5 hours), break it into chunks (makes 24 bites).

There are approximately 117 Calories per bite: 2.4g Protein; 3.3g Carbohydrate; 10.2g Fat; and 1.2g Dietary Fibre. The following table shows the percentage (%) of RDI/AI in each Chocky Nutty Roadblock bite.

Gender and Age Group	Essential Vitamins				Essential Minerals (and Iron)					
	A	B2	B3	E	CALC	MAG	PHOS	POT	SOD*	IRON
Male >30/>50 years	18	6	2	21	3	12/11	5	4	5	12
Female >30/>50 years	23	7	2	30	3	15	5	5	5	5/12

*based on lowest daily AI

Each Chocky Nutty Roadblock bite contains 1% or less of the RDI/AI for vitamins B1, B5, B6, B7(0%), B9, B12, C(0%), D(0%) and K, for both males and females for the selected age groups.

Chocolate Coated Maple balls

These are so delicious it is hard to believe that they are a healthy snack. They make a wonderful afternoon treat, or desert after a light evening meal. The biggest challenge is only eating one!

You will need:
150g roasted almonds
150g roasted cashews
60g honey
25g maple syrup
¼ tsp salt
80g dark chocolate (70-85%) (use carob for a vegan option)
86g chocolate protein powder

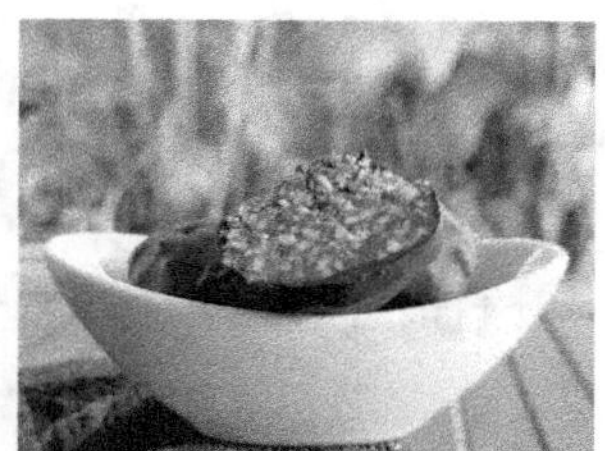

How to make them:
1) Place the almonds and cashews in a food processor and blend at high speed until they resemble a coarse flour consistency.
2) Add the remaining ingredients and blend on a low speed until you have a fine, sticky crumb.
3) Shape the mixture into small balls and place the balls into the fridge for 1-2 hours until they are set hard (if you are short for time pop them in a freezer for about 30 minutes).
3) Melt the dark chocolate, and dip each ball into the chocolate to coat.
4) Place the balls onto a tray lined with baking paper and put them back into the fridge to set.
5) Serve. Eat. Enjoy.
There are approximately 138 calories per ball: 6g Protein; 10g Carbohydrate; 9g Fat; and 2g Dietary Fibre. The following table shows the percentage (%) of RDI/AI in each Chocolate Coated Maple ball.

Gender and Age Group	Essential Vitamins											Essential Minerals (and Iron)					
	A	B1	B2	B3	B5	B6	B9	B12	C	E	K	CALC	MAG	PHOS	POT	SOD*	IRON
Male >30/>50 years	4	4	7	2	2	3/2	1	7	3	24	7	6	15	12	5	9	17
Female >30/>50 years	6	4	8	3	3	3	1	7	3	34	8	6	20/19	12	6	9	7/17

*based on lowest daily AI

Each Chocolate Coated Maple balls contains 1% or less of the RDI/ AI for vitamins B7(0%), B9, and D(0%) for both males and females for the selected age groups.

Oven-baked Snacks

The snacks in this section need baking, so you will need access to an oven to make them. However, once made the snacks can be stored in containers and are just as accessible as the snacks made without an oven.

Vegetable chips

Make your own vegetable chips if you want to know the amount and type of oil or salt used in preparing and cooking them. Sweet potato and beetroot chips can be used to add to your vegetable intake.

How to make chips:
1) Preheat oven to 200°C.
2) Finely slice the sweet potato and/or beetroot as thin as you can get them (approx 2-3 mm).
3) Lay the slices on a baking tray, and sprinkle with salt
4) Bake in the oven until crispy (Approx 20-25 minutes but the time will depend on the thickness of the slices).
5) Allow to cool and then put them in a well-sealed bag/container ready for the road!

Carrot Chips

Carrots are great because they can be sweet or spicy. Sprinkle brown sugar over them for a sweeter chip. For spicy chips add a light dusting of curry powder, or spices (e.g. Mediterranean spice mix, cayenne pepper) to make your carrot chips a more exciting snack.

Zucchini chips

Zucchinis can be used to make vegetable chips. Season them to taste with salt, pepper or parmesan cheese before baking.

Apple chips

The sweetness of apple chips is influenced by the type of apple you choose. Sprinkle thinly sliced apple pieces with cinnamon sugar (and/or brown sugar) before baking for an apple pie taste.

Vegetable Chips	Essential Vitamins													Essential Minerals and Iron					
	A	B1	B2	B3	B5	B6	B 7	B9	B12	C	D	E	K	CALC	MAG	PHOS	POT	SOD	IRON
Sweet potato	●					●		●		●		●					●	●	
Beetroot		●	●	●				●		●				●			●	●	
Carrot	●	●	●	●	●	●		●		●		●	●	●	●	●	●	●	
Zucchini	●	●	●	●	●	●		●		●		●	●	●	●	●	●	●	
Apple	●	●	●	●	●	●		●		●		●	●	●	●	●	●	●	

Get me out of this Jam Square

These squares are really sweet. If you do not have a sweet tooth, use a tart jam to reduce the sweetness. Alternatively, add natural yoghurt to offset the sweetness for a delicious more substantial snack. If you are looking for a sweet snack, this is a good option.

What you need:
120g unsalted butter
100g almond butter
4 tbsp maple syrup
150g rolled oats
120g almond flour
100g coconut flour
90g brown sugar
1 tsp baking powder
½ tsp sea salt
½ tsp vanilla extract
½ tsp ground cinnamon
340g strawberry jam (you can use any jam)
1 tsp lemon juice

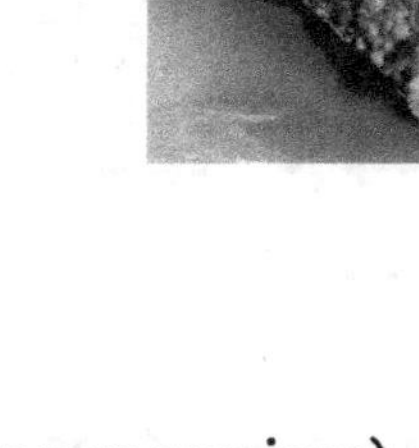

How to make them:
1) Preheat oven to 180°C. Line a 23cm x 23cm tray with baking paper
2) Combine the butter, almond butter, and maple syrup in a bowl and mix well.
3) Add the rolled oats, almond flour, coconut flour, sugar, baking powder, salt, vanilla extract, and cinnamon to the butter mixture and stir until it makes a soft dough. Then, put aside one third of the dough mix.
4) Put the dough onto the baking paper and press spreading the dough evenly in the tray.
5) Combine the jam, lemon juice, and salt in a small bowl. Then spread the jam mixture evenly over the dough in the tray.
6) Crumble the remaining dough over the jam mixture, then press down trapping the jam between the layers.

7) Bake in the oven until it is golden brown (approximately 35-40 minutes).

8) Once it has cooled, cut into 18 squares and store in an air tight container.

There are approximately 257 calories per Jam Square: 5.1 Protein; 29.3 Carbohydrate; 13.1g Fat; and 3.3g Dietary Fibre. The following table shows the percentage (%) of RDI/AI in each Jam Square.

Gender and Age Group	Essential Vitamins								Essential Minerals (and Iron)					
	A	B1	B2	B3	B5	B9	C	E	CALC	MAG	PHOS	POT	SOD*	IRON
Male >30/>50 years	20	4	4	2	2	2	8	10	5	7/6	8	8	2	14
Female >30/>50 years	25	4	4	2	3	2	8	14	5	9/8	8	11	2	6/14

*based on lowest daily AI

Each Jam Square contains 1% or less of the RDI/AI for vitamins B6, B7(0%), B12, D(0%) and K for both males and females for the selected age groups.

Crunchy Road Bars

These crunchy bars are similar to store bought muesli bars, without all the hidden surprises. It is a snack filled with dietary fibre and is not as sweet as the other bars. It is a great snack to take with you on the road.

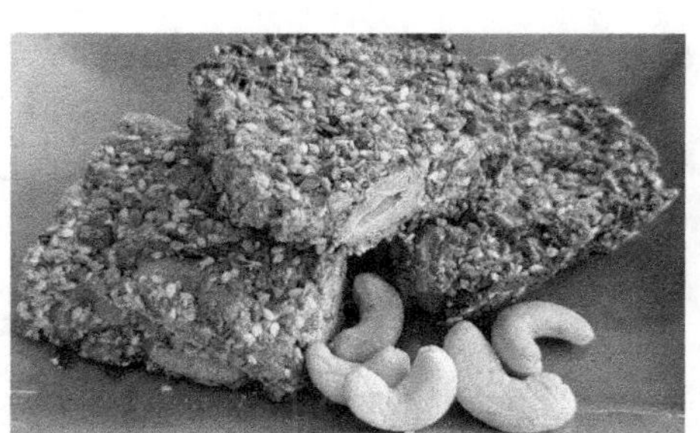

What you need:
300g cashews
100g maple syrup
50g wheat bran
8 tbsp (6 + 2) raw sesame seeds
6 tbsp (5 + 1) flaxseed
¼ tsp ground cinnamon (or cardamom)
¾ tsp sea salt
1 tbsp coconut oil

How to make them:
1) Heat the over to (200°C).
2) Line a 23cm x 23cm tray with baking paper
3) Put half of the cashews, 6 tablespoons of the sesame seeds, and 5 tablespoons of the flaxseed in the oven (200°C) to toast, until golden brown (approx 10-12 minutes). They may need to be stirred occasionally.
4) Then, leave to cool down. Put oven down to 180°C
5) Put 2 tbsp sesame seeds and 1 tbsp flaxseed aside.
6) Combine cashews and remaining sesame and flaxseeds with the wheat bran, salt, and ground cinnamon and process until finely chopped.
7) Put the maple syrup and coconut oil into a saucepan and bring to the boil, then gently stir for 1 minute.
8) Pour the maple syrup mixture over the cashew mixture and stir to coat.
9) Put the combined mixture in the baking tray and press down firmly until it is evenly spread. The mixture will be sticky, when you are pressing it.

10) Bake for 25–30 minutes until it is golden brown
11) Wait until the mixture is very cool (at least one hour) before cutting into 18 squares. When the bars are completely cold, they can be stored in an air tight container.

There are approximately 171 calories per bar: 4.7g Protein; 8.6g Carbohydrate; 13.1g Fat; and 3.7g Dietary Fibre. The following table shows the percentage (%) of RDI/AI contained in each Crunchy Road Bar.

Gender and Age Group	Essential Vitamins								Essential Minerals (and Iron)					
	B1	B2	B3	B5	B6	B9	E	K	CALC	MAG	PHOS	POT	SOD*	IRON
Male >30/>50 years	19	2	4	4	11/9	5	2	8	6	21/20	17	5	22	27
Female >30/>50 years	21	3	5	6	11/10	5	2	10	6	27/26	17	7	22	12/27

*based on lowest daily AI

Each Crunchy Road Bar contains 1% or less of the RDI/AI for vitamins A, B7(0%), B12(0%), C, and D(0%) for both males and females for the selected age groups.

Cherry Seed Squares

These squares are chewy, and go well with a cuppa!

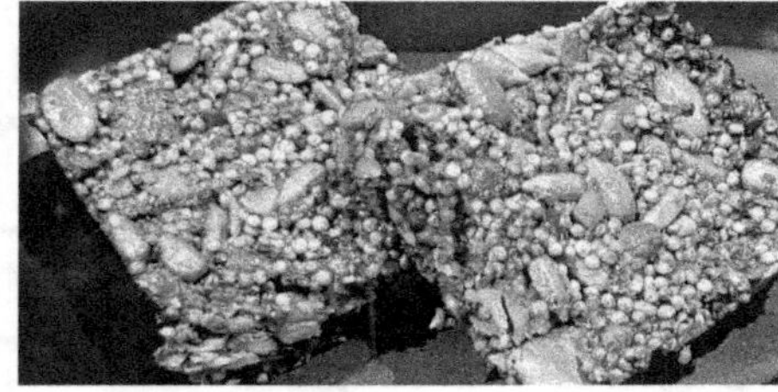

What you need:
200g chopped almonds
100g raw quinoa
25g raw pumpkin seeds
25g raw sunflower seeds
100g dried cherries
(can be substituted with glacè cherries)
2 tbsp maple syrup (substitute with honey if preferred)
¾ tsp sea salt
2 tbsp water

How to make them:
1) Line a 23cm x 23cm tray with baking paper.
2) Set the oven temperature to 180°C.
3) Toast chopped almonds, raw quinoa, pumpkin seeds, and sunflower seeds in the oven, stirring until golden brown (approximately 10-12 minutes). Leave to cool.
4) Process the cherries, maple syrup, salt and water in a food processor until smooth.
5) Put in a bowl with the toasted almond mixture from the oven and mix well.
6) Press firmly in the tray until it is evenly spread.
7) Bake for 20–25 minutes (until it is no longer sticky)
8) Leave it to cool down and then cut into 16 bars.
9) When the bars are completely cold, they can be stored in an air tight container.

There are approximately 134 calories per bar: 4g Protein; 10.1g Carbohydrate; 8.4g Fat; and 1.8g Dietary Fibre. The following table shows the percentage (%) of RDI/AI in each Cherry Seed Square.

Gender and Age Group	Essential Vitamins								Essential Minerals (and Iron)				
	A	B1	B2	B3	B5	B6	B9	E	MAG	PHOS	POT	SOD*	IRON
Male >30/>50 years	2	8	2	3	1	6/5	4	21	5	4	1	24	5
Female >30/>50 years	3	9	2	4	2	6/5	4	30	7	4	2	24	2/5

*based on lowest daily AI

Each Cherry Seed Square contains 1% or less of the RDI/AI for vitamins B7(0%), B12(0%), C, D(0%), K, and calcium for both males and females for the selected age groups. Also, it contains 1% or less of the RDI/AI for vitamin B5 and potassium for men.

Nutty Mud Cookies

These banana and peanut cookies are a satisfying snack, and go well with your morning tea.

What you need:
180g rolled oats
50g pecans
1 medium carrot (grated)
3 large bananas
25g pumpkin seeds, unsalted and raw
25g sultanas
120g peanut butter
1 tsp ground cinnamon

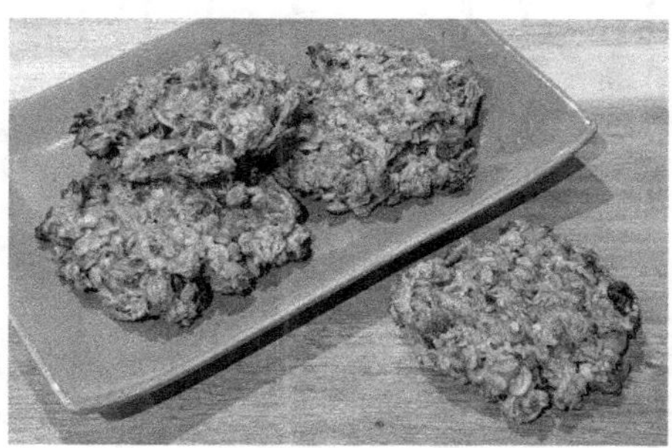

How to make them:
1) Preheat oven to 180°C.
2) Line a tray with baking
3) Grate the carrot, and mash the bananas
4) Mix together the oats, cinnamon, banana, and peanut butter. Add the grated carrot, pumpkin seeds, pecans and sultanas. Mix well.
5) Roll into balls, and put them on the lined tray, then press down to form a cookie shape (makes 18 cookies).
6) Bake for approximately 15 minutes until golden brown.
7) Remove from oven and leave to cool. When cooled store in an airtight container.

There are approximately 104 calories per cookie: 3.3g Protein; 11.5g Carbohydrate; 4.9g Fat; and 2.0g Dietary Fibre. The following table shows the percentage (%) of RDI/AI of each nutrient in a Nutty Mud Cookie.

Gender and Age Group	Essential Vitamins										Essential Minerals (and Iron)					
	A	B1	B2	B3	B5	B6	B9	C	E	K	CALC	MAG	PHOS	POT	SOD*	IRON
Male >30/>50 years	76	6	4	7	5	9/7	4	5	5	3	3	10	7	5	7	11
Female >30/>50 years	98	7	4	8	7	9/7	4	5	8	3	3	13	7	7	7	5/11

*based on lowest daily AI

Each Nutty Mud Cookie contains 1% or less of the RDI/AI for vitamins B7(0%), B12(0%), and D(0%) for both males and females for the selected age groups. Also, one cookie contains 98% of the RDI for vitamin A for women.

Cranberry Country Squares

These squares are delicious, they are not as sweet as the Cherry Seed Squares but a little sweeter than the Crunchy Road Bars.

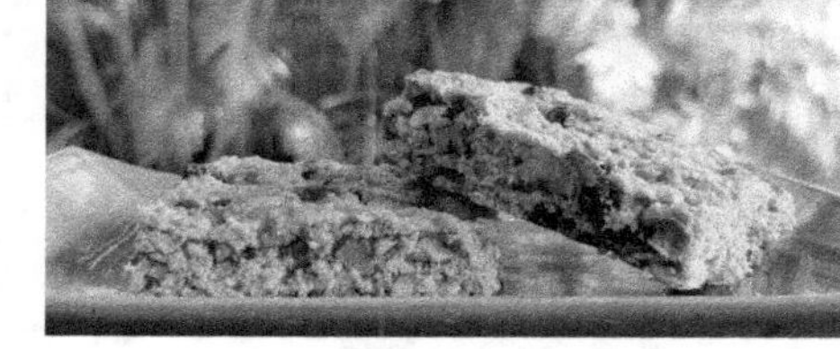

What you need:
300g rolled oats
140g unsalted butter
200g brown sugar
2 large eggs
2 tbsps milk
½ tsp nutmeg
½ tsp baking soda
200g plain flour (or all-purpose flour for gluten-free)
150g chopped pecans
170g dried cranberries

How to make them:
1) Preheat oven to 200°C.
2) Line a 25 x 25cm baking tray.
3) Toast the oats on a tray in the oven until they are golden (approximately 15 minutes). Then, reduce the oven to 180°C
4) Combine the butter and sugar and mix until fluffy. Add eggs, milk, and mix well.
5) Add flour, nutmeg and baking soda, then mix into the butter mixture.
6) Add the oats, chopped pecans, and cranberries.
7) Spread the mixture in the tray, press down firmly and bake for 25 minutes (until golden).
8 Cool, then cut into 24 squares (or 32 squares).
You can reduce the amount of calories you are consuming by cutting into smaller squares. This recipe makes 24 squares (approx 6x6cm) and can quite easily be cut into 32 slightly smaller squares which reduces each square by approximately 60 calories.

When cut into 24 squares, there are approximately 229 calories per square: 3.6g Protein; 28.4g Carbohydrate; 11.2g Fat; and 1.0g

Dietary. The following table shows the percentage (%) of RDI/AI in each Cranberry Country Square when cut into 24 squares.

Gender and Age Group	Essential Vitamins											Essential Minerals (and Iron)					
	A	B1	B2	B3	B5	B6	B9	B12	D	E	K	CALC	MAG	PHOS	POT	SOD*	IRON
Male >30/>50 years	22	13	7	5	5	2	6	3	47/23	3	1	4	8/7	8	3	3	16
Female >30/>50 years	28	14	8	5	7	2	6	3	47/23	4	1	4	10	9	4	3	7/16

*based on lowest daily AI

Each Cranberry Country Square contains 1% or less of the RDI/AI for vitamins B7(0%) and C for both males and females for the selected age groups. One square contains 1% or less of the AI for vitamin K for men.

When cut into 32 squares, there are approximately 172 calories per square: 2.7g Protein; 21.3g Carbohydrate; 8.4g Fat; and 0.8g Dietary Fibre. The following table shows the percentage (%) of RDI/AI in each Cranberry Country Square when cut into 32 squares.

Gender and Age Group	Essential Vitamins											Essential Minerals (and Iron)					
	A	B1	B2	B3	B5	B6	B9	B12	D	E	K	CALC	MAG	PHOS	POT	SOD*	IRON
Male >30/>50 years	17	10	5	4	4	2/1	4	2	35/18	2	1	3	6/5	7	2	2	12
Female >30/>50 years	21	10	6	4	5	2/1	4	2	35/18	3	1	3	7	7	3	2	5/12

*based on lowest daily AI

Each Cranberry Country Square contains 1% or less of the RDI/AI for vitamins B7(0%) and C for both males and females for the selected age groups. One square contains 1% or less of the AI for vitamin K for women.

CHAPTER FIVE: ELECTRICAL EQUIPMENT REQUIRED

Making your own snacks means that you can control what goes in to the snack, making sure that they are packed full of nutritional benefits, and contain less fillers and chemicals. Many of the ideas in the next section contain nuts and seeds, providing a good amount of healthy fats, and natural protein. Protein powder can also be added to most of the snacks.

Food processor favourites

These recipes require a food processor to chop and combine the ingredients into a paste. Most of them can be made with a small 1 cup mini food processor, a small appliance that is portable so there is no need for large expensive appliances to make the balls and squares.

Bumpy Road Bliss Balls

These snacks are not only for eating on bumpy roads, you can snack on them anytime!

You will need:
100g pitted dates
200g roasted almonds
4 tbsp natural peanut butter
1 tbsp cacao powder
Water (1-3 tablespoons if needed)
Crushed peanuts to decorate balls (optional).

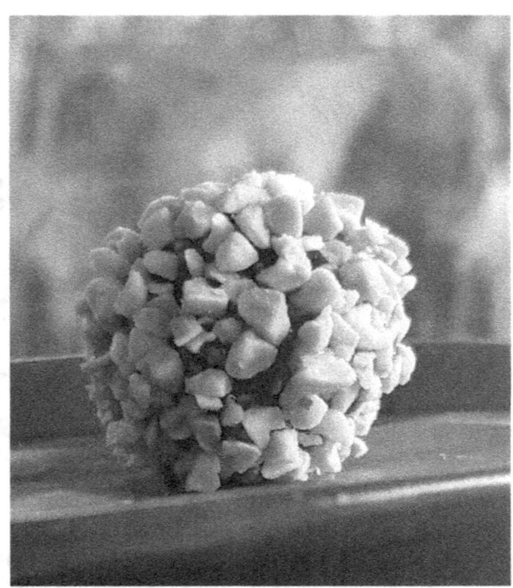

How to make them:
1) Put all of the ingredients into a food processor and blend. The mixture should feel a little sticky so add water if it is a bit too dry.
2) Shape the mixture in snack-sized balls, and then roll them in crushed peanuts (makes 14 balls).
3) Place the balls on a baking paper lined tray and refrigerate for 30 minutes. Store in an air tight container.

There are approximately 153 calories in each ball: 4.7g Protein; 7.0g Carbohydrate; 11.5g Fat; and 1.7g Dietary Fibre. The following table shows the percentage (%) of RDI/AI in each Bumpy Road Bliss Ball.

Gender and Age Group	Essential Vitamins									Essential Minerals (and Iron)					
	A	B1	B2	B3	B5	B6	B9	B12	E	CALC	MAG	PHOS	POT	SOD*	IRON
Male >30/>50 years	2	3	12	8	3	4/3	3	2	41	5	13	10	5	6	9
Female >30/>50 years	3	4	14	9	5	4/3	3	2	59	5	17	10	7	6	4/9

*based on lowest daily AI

Each Bumpy Road Bliss Ball contains 1% or less of the RDI/AI for vitamins B7(0%), C and K for both males and females for the selected age groups.

Lonely Peak Pistachio Protein balls

These chocolatey balls are so much fun with their bright green nutty coating.

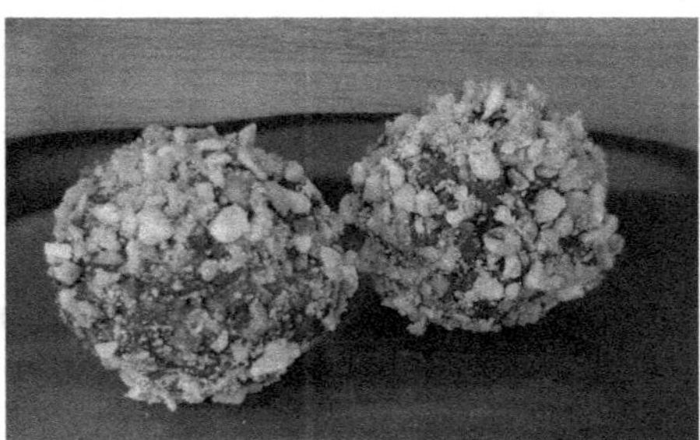

You will need:
125g pistachio nuts (shells removed)
40g finely chopped dark chocolate (85-92%)
1 tbsp coconut flour
1 tbsp protein powder
25g cacao powder
85g almond paste or almond butter
80g maple syrup (honey can be used as a substitute)
Extra pistachio nuts to decorate the balls (optional)

How to make them:
1) Finely chop the 125g pistachios and put aside. Finely chop or grind extra pistachio nuts.
2) Put the 125g chopped pistachios into a bowl and add the remaining dry ingredients. Mix well.
3) Add the remaining ingredients and mix until it is the right consistency to roll into balls. If it is too dry add more syrup, and if it is too wet, add more flour or protein powder.
4) Shape into balls, roll in the crushed pistachio nuts, and place on a tray lined with baking paper (makes approximately 16 balls).
5) Place in the refrigerator to set.

There are approximately 103 calories per ball: 4.1g Protein; 4.8g Carbohydrate; 7.5g Fat; and 2.4g Dietary Fibre. The following table shows the percentage (%) of RDI/AI in each Lonely Peak Pistachio Protein Ball.

Gender and Age Group	Essential Vitamins						Essential Minerals (and Iron)					
	A	B2	B12	C	E	K	CALC	MAG	PHOS	POT	SOD*	IRON
Male >30/>50 years	1	1	2	1	1	1	2	5	2	2	1	4
Female >30/>50 years	2	1	2	1	1	1	2	7/6	2	2	1	2/4

*based on lowest daily AI

Each Lonely Peak Pistachio Protein Ball contains 1% or less of the RDI/AI for vitamins B1, B2, B3, B5, B6, B7 (0%), B9, C, D(0%), E and K; and sodium (based on the lowest daily AI), for both males and females for the selected age groups.

Red Rock Protein Balls

These stunning red balls are a great treat. It might be hard to find freeze-dried raspberry powder in remote area so they can be eaten without it but if you can coat the balls in bright red raspberry powder it is worth the effort.

What you need:
100g pitted dates
75g walnuts
75g hazelnuts
2 tbsp chocolate protein powder
1 tsp cacao powder
1 tbsp coconut oil (melted)
Water (1-3 tablespoons if needed)
Freeze-dried raspberries to decorate balls

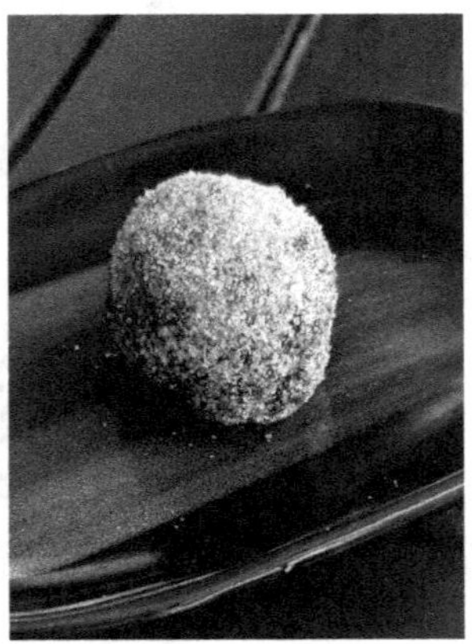

How to make them:
1) Put the dates, walnuts and hazelnuts in a food processor and blend.
2) Add the protein powder, cacao powder and coconut oil and blend again until mixed well. The mixture should feel a little sticky (add water if it is too dry).
3) Crush the freeze-dried raspberries, and put the powder on a plate or flat surface.
4) Shape the mix into snack sized balls, roll in the raspberry powder and place the balls on a baking paper lined tray (makes approximately 14 balls).
5) Place in the fridge to set (approximately 1 hour). Store them in an airtight container.
There are approximately 114 calories per ball: 2.2g Protein; 7g Carbohydrate; 8.3g Fat; and 1.1g Dietary Fibre. The following table shows the percentage (%) of RDI/AI in each Red Rock Protein Ball (%).

Gender and Age Group	Essential Vitamins											Essential Minerals (and Iron)				
	A	B1	B2	B3	B5	B6	B9	B12	C	E	K	CALC	MAG	PHOS	POT	IRON
Male >30/>50 years	3	5	2	2	2	6/4	3	2	2	9	2	3	7	5	4	7
Female >30/>50 years	3	5	2	2	3	6/5	3	2	2	13	3	3	9	5	5	3/7

Each Red Rock Protein Ball contains 1% or less of the RDI/AI for vitamins B7 and D(0%), and sodium (based on the lowest daily AI), for both males and females for the selected age groups.

Outback Apricot Balls

The apricot, cashew and coconut combination makes for a great snack.

What you need:
100g dried apricots
40g walnuts
50g cashews
2 tbsp coconut oil
1 tsp ground ginger
50g desiccated coconut

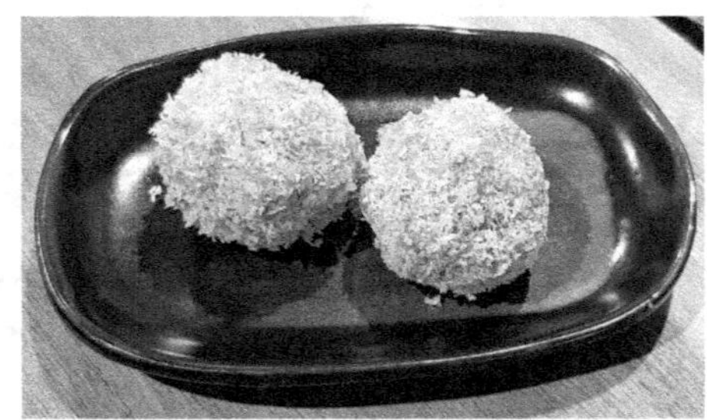

Garnish with desiccated coconut.

How to make them:
1) Place the dried apricots, walnuts and cashews in a food processor and blend.
2) Add the coconut oil, ground ginger and desiccated coconut and blend. The mixture should feel a little sticky. If the mixture feels a bit dry, add a little more coconut oil.
3) Roll the mixture into snack-sized balls and place on the tray lined with baking paper (makes approximately 10 balls).
4) Put the extra desiccated coconut onto a plate or flat surface and roll the balls to coat.
5) Refrigerate the balls for 30 minutes to set.
6) Store them in an airtight container.

There are approximately 151 calories per ball: 2.3g Protein; 6.1g Carbohydrate; 12.8g Fat; and 2g Dietary Fibre. The following table shows the percentage (%) of RDI/AI in each Outback Apricot Ball.

Gender and Age Group	Essential Vitamins									Essential Minerals (and Iron)			
	B1	B2	B5	B6	B7	B12	D	E	K	MAG	PHOS	POT	IRON
Male >30/>50 years	3	18	2	4/3	3	4	7/4	3	9	7	14	2	7
Female >30/>50 years	4	21	3	4/3	4	4	7/4	5	10	9	14	2	3/7

Each Outback Apricot Ball contains 1% or less of the RDI/AI for vitamins A, B3, B9 and C, calcium, and sodium (based on the lowest daily AI), for both males and females for the selected age groups.

Salted Creek Stones

These balls get their natural sweetness from the dates.

What you need:
80g pitted dates
200g macadamia nuts (extra to decorate (optional))
75g almond butter (or paste)
1 tbsp coconut oil (liquid)
1 tsp sea salt
1-2 tbsp water (as needed)

How to make them:
1) Place the dates, macadamia nuts and almond butter in a food processor and blend until combined.
2) Add the coconut oil and sea salt and blend into a dough. The mixture should feel a little sticky.
3) Shape the mixture into balls and roll in the crushed macadamia nuts (makes approximately 12 balls).
4) Refrigerate the balls for 30 minutes to set. Store.

There are approximately 205 calories per ball: 8.3g Protein; 38.4g Carbohydrate; 1.9g Fat; 3.3g Dietary Fibre. The following table shows the percentage (%) of RDI/AI in each Salted Creek Stone.

Gender and Age Group	Essential Vitamins					Essential Minerals (and Iron)					
	B1	B2	B3	B5	B6	CALC	MAG	PHOS	POT	SOD*	IRON
Male >30/>50 years	18	5	4	3	5/4	3	9	5	4	32	10
Female >30/>50 years	19	6	5	5	5	3	12/11	5	5	32	5/10

*based on lowest daily AI

Each Salted Creek Stone has 1% or less of the RDI/AI for vitamins A, B7(0%), B9, B12(0%), C, D(0%), E, and K for both males and females for the selected age groups.

Roadtrip Bliss Bites

These are just as good made into bites or balls – it is up to you!

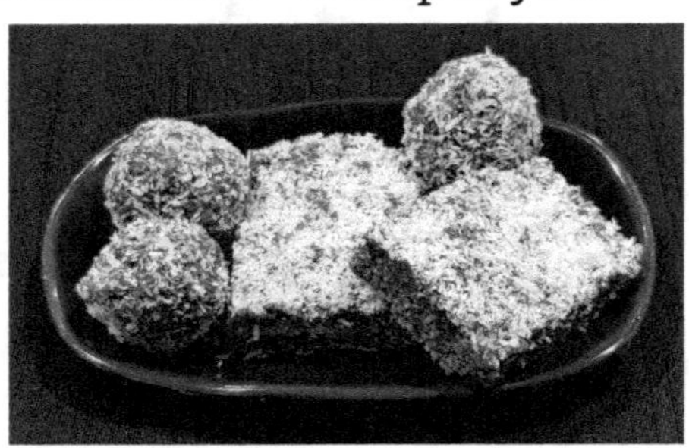

What you need:
120g pitted dates
100g almond meal
80g chocolate protein powder
45g desiccated coconut, plus
  extra for rolling
Desiccated coconut or crushed
peanuts to decorate

How to make them:
1) Line a 23 x 23cm baking tray with baking paper.
2) Put the dates in a bowl and cover with boiling water - leave to soak for 30 minutes, then drain.
3) Place the almond meal, dates, protein powder and coconut in a food processor or high-powered blender and process until well combined. Ensure everything is well mixed.
4) The mixture should be a little sticky, but if it is too thick, try adding some water.
5) Put the mixture into the tray and press firmly.
6) Sprinkle the desiccated coconut over the mixture before placing in a cool place (fridge is best) for 30 minutes).
7) Once firm, cut into 12 squares and store in an airtight container.

There are approximately 111 calories per bite: 6.2g Protein; 10g Carbohydrate; 4.7g Fat; and 1.3g Dietary Fibre. The following table shows the percentage (%) of RDI/AI in each Roadtrip Bliss Bite.

Gender and Age Group	Essential Vitamins							Essential Minerals (and Iron)					
	A	B5	B6	B12	C	E	K	CALC	MAG	PHOS	POT	SOD*	IRON
Male >30/>50 years	10	2	2	13	7	7	6	7	11	7	5	7	12
Female >30/>50 years	12	2	2	13	7	10	7	7	15/14	7	7	7	5/12

*based on lowest daily AI

Each Roadtrip Bliss bite (or ball) contains 1% or less of the RDI/AI for vitamins B1, B2, B3, B7(0%), B9, and D(0%), E, and K for both males and females for the selected age groups.

Oh fudge, these are good balls!

Oh fudge, these are good balls are a healthy snack, with the added nutrition of the super food chia to make them extra nutritious!

What you need:
220g dates
85g chia seeds
50g almonds
2 tbsps cacao
Seasalt salt (optional)
1 tbsp coconut oil (if needed)

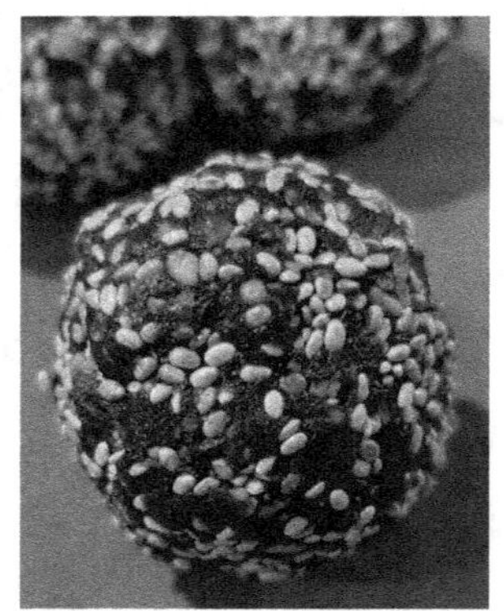

The almonds can be substituted with hazelnuts, walnuts or pecans.

How to make them:
1) Add chia seeds to the food processor and pulse a few times. Chop it finer for smoother balls.
2) Add the remaining ingredients and mix on low speed for 2-3 minutes. The mixture should resemble dough, so process for longer if needed.
3) Add small amounts of water or coconut oil slowly if the mixture is too dry.
4) Once you have sticky dough, shape it into small balls (makes approximately 20).
5) Place the balls on the lined baking tray and leave to set. Store in an airtight container.

There are approximately 79 calories per ball: 2.2g Protein; 8.5g Carbohydrate; 3.8g Fat; and 3.2g Dietary Fibre. The following table shows the percentage (%) of RDI/AI in each Oh Fudge! Ball.

Gender and Age Group	Essential Vitamins							Essential Minerals (and Iron)				
	A	B1	B2	B3	B5	B6	E	CALC	MAG	PHOS	POT	IRON
Male >30/>50 years	2	1	3	2	2	2/1	7	5	7	6	4	7
Female >30/>50 years	2	2	3	2	3	2	9	5	10/9	6	5	3/7

Each Oh Fudge! Ball contains 1% or less of the RDI/AI for vitamins A (males only), B7(0%), B9, B12(0%), C(0%), D(0%) and K, and sodium (based on the lowest daily AI), for both males and females for the selected age groups.

Get me through the Afternoon Energy Bites

Sometimes you just need something to get your through the afternoon. Before you reach for a high carbohydrate snack, consider these protein rich bites as a healthier alternative.

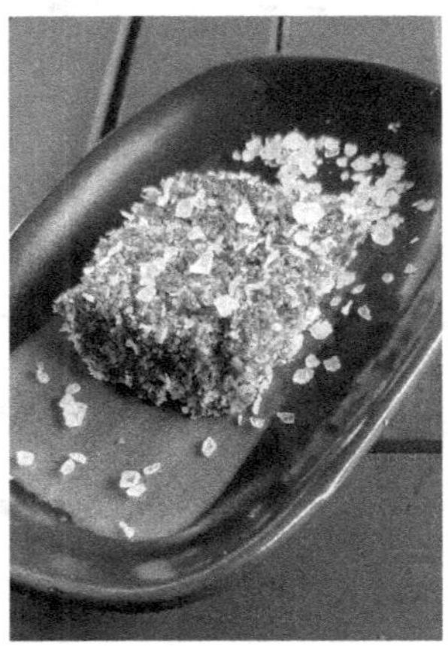

What you need:
1 tbsp coconut oil
3 tbsp cacao
140g pitted dates (about 8)
100g nut butter
3 tbsp ground chia seeds
1 tsp sea salt
½ tsp ground cinnamon
3 tbsp almond flour or meal
3 tbsp desiccated coconut

How to make it:
1) Line a 23 x 23cm tray with baking paper.
2) Put dates in a small bowl and cover with boiling water. Leave for 10 minutes, then drain.
3) Put dates, nut butter and oil into the food processor and process until ingredients combine into a crumbly mixture.
4) Add chia seeds, salt, and cinnamon. Mix well.
6) Add almond flour, cacao, and desiccated coconut, and process to combine.
7) Press the mixture into the tray pressing as firmly as possible (mix will look slightly greasy).
8) Cover and leave to firm (if you have a refrigerator it will take about 1 hour). It will take longer without a refrigerator, depending on the room temperature in your climate.
9) Once firm, cut into 18 squares, and sprinkle with sea salt (optional).
10) Store in an airtight container.

There are approximately 101 calories per square: 2.8g Protein; 7.8g Carbohydrate; 6.4g Fat; and 1.9g Dietary Fibre. The following table shows the percentage (%) of RDI/AI in each Afternoon Energy Bite.

Gender and Age Group	Essential Vitamins					Essential Minerals (and Iron)					
	A	B2	B3	B5	B6	CALC	MAG	PHOS	POT	SOD*	IRON
Male >30/>50 years	1	3	2	2	2	5	13/12	5	5	29	12
Female >30/>50 years	2	4	2	2	2	5	17/16	5	7	29	5/12

*based on lowest daily AI

Each Afternoon Energy Bite contains 1% or less of the RDI/AI for vitamins A (males only), B1, B7(0%), B9, B12(0%), C, D(0%), E and K, for both males and females for the selected age groups.

These bite back!

The name says it all. These bites will be the snack of choice for those looking for a snack with a spicier edge! The nutrients have been calculated based on cutting the dough into 18 or 24 squares. Choose your bite size!

What you need:
70g walnuts
70g desiccated coconut
200g pitted dates, roughly chopped
1 tsp ground tumeric
½ tsp ground cinnamon
1 tbsp unsweetened cocoa powder
1 scoop (approx 40g) chocolate protein powder

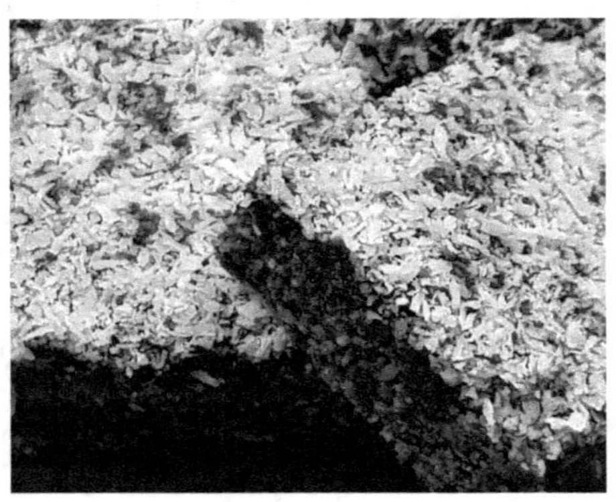

How to make them:
1) Line a 23 x 23cm baking tray with baking paper.
2) Roughly chop the walnuts and dates.
3) Put all of the ingredients in a food processor and pulse until the dates and walnuts are in small pieces and the mixture sticks together (add more dates if the mixture is too dry).
4) Press the mixture in the baking paper lined tray and leave to set. Cut into bite sized pieces.

If you make 18 bites, there are approximately 97 calories per square: 1.7g Protein; 9.6g Carbohydrate; 5.5g Fat; and 1.3g Dietary Fibre. The following table shows the percentage (%) of RDI/AI in each piece of These Bite Back when making 18 squares.

Gender and Age Group	Essential Vitamins											Essential Minerals (and Iron)					
	A	B1	B2	B3	B5	B6	B9	B12	C	E	K	CALC	MAG	PHOS	POT	SOD*	IRON
Male >30/>50 years	4	2	2	2	2	4/3	2	4	2	2	2	4	10	4	5	2	10
Female >30/>50 years	6	2	2	2	4	4	2	4	2	3	3	4	13	4	7	2	5/10

*based on lowest daily AI

Each These Bite Back contains 1% or less of the RDI/AI for vitamins B7 and D(0%) for both males and females for the selected age groups.

If you make 24 bites, there are approximately 74 calories per square: 1.3g Protein; 7.4g Carbohydrate; 4.2g Fat; and 1g Dietary Fibre. The following table shows the percentage (%) of RDI/AI in each piece of These Bite Back when making 24 squares.

Gender and Age Group	Essential Vitamins											Essential Minerals (and Iron)					
	A	B1	B2	B3	B5	B6	B9	B12	C	E	K	CALC	MAG	PHOS	POT	SOD*	IRON
Male >30/>50 years	3	2	1	1	2	3/2	1	3	2	2	2	3	8/7	3	4	2	7.5
Female >30/>50 years	4	2	2	1	3	3	1	3	2	2	2	3	10	3	5	3	3/8

*based on lowest daily AI

CHAPTER SIX: DRINKS

Drinks are another good way to increase your nutrient intake. This section contains suggestions on ways to include nutrient rich drinks in your day!

Lemon and Ginger tea
Combine lemon with ginger root to make this refreshing lemon and ginger tea. Sweeten with honey if needed.

What you need:
½ - 1 lemon (to taste)
2cm piece ginger root
Pure Honey

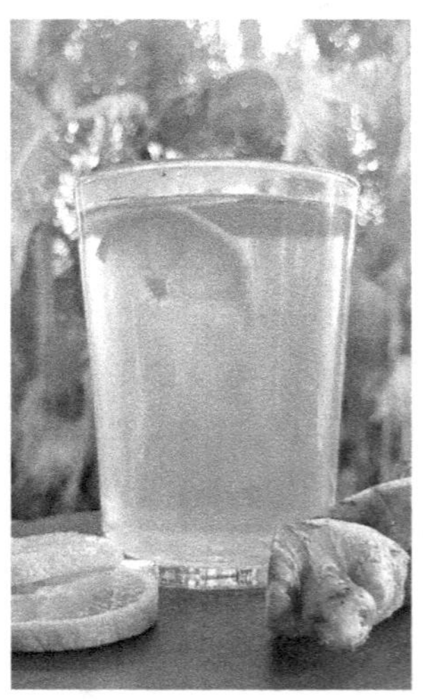

How to make hot tea:
1) Cut the lemon in half. Squeeze the juice from one half and slice the rest.
2) Put the lemon juice in a glass along with slices of the finely sliced ginger.
3) Fill with boiling water and leave to steep for 3 minutes or until cool enough to sip.
4) Sweeten with honey (to taste). Make sure it is 'real' honey not a sugar substitute.

Ginger and lemon tea can also be made into a cold refreshing drink.

How to make iced tea:
1) Make as per the previous instructions using a 700ml glass bot-

tle, adjusting the quantities to your taste.

2) Let the lemon and ginger steep in the boiling water, add some honey while it is still warm and then let it cool. Once cool, put in the fridge to chill. Add ice (if available) for individual cold drinks.

ESSENTIAL VITAMINS													ESSENTIAL MINERALS					
A	B1	B2	B3	B5	B6	B 7	B9	B12	C	D	E	K	CALC	MAG	PHOS	POT	SOD	IRON
●							●		●				●	●		●	●	●

Better with a blender

Smoothies are a great way to consume nutrients in one tasty drink. While fresh is always best, if you are short on time in the mornings, you can make your smoothies the night before or store the ingredients in bags ready to blend. If you prepare the night before, chop all the ingredients and then put them in bags measured for one smoothie. If possible put them in the freezer (this will create a thicker smoothie and anything that should not go into a freezer (e.g. leafy greens) in the fridge. If you do not have access to a freezer, put everything in the fridge. The next morning, simply put everything into your blender, and you can have breakfast on-the-move.

While smoothies always taste better when they are freshly blended, they can be made the day before if more convenient. Please be aware that some flavours may change. Add a squeeze of lemon or lime to stop it from going brown.

Foods that improve the nutrient density include:
- Fruit: You can add other soft fruit, e.g. strawberries, blueberries or whole fruit such as mango which does not need refrigeration until it has been cut.
- Spirulina: Add 1 tsp of spirulina to increase the nutrient density of the smoothie considerably.
- Psyllium husks: Add 1 tbsp of psyllium husks to add more dietary fibre (if you add psyllium do not leave it too long before you drink the smoothie because the psyllium will expand and it may become too thick to drink.

Fruit and Veg Smoothie

Smoothies are an easy, convenient and nutritious but sometimes too much fruit can increase blood sugar levels. Smoothies with a combination of fruit and vegetables usually have lower levels of sugar, are just as easy to make.

What you need:
½ mango
1 kiwi fruit
1 small stalk of celery (including the leaves)
1 small Lebanese cucumber
½ bunch of bok choy
½ tbsp of maca powder
½ tbsp of chia seeds
200ml Coconut water

How to make it:
1) Chop up the mango, kiwi fruit and greens. Blend.
2) Add the maca powder, chia seeds and coconut water (the amount of coconut water added will determine the thickness of the smoothie). Blend until smooth

There are approximately 221 calories in the Fruit and Veg Smoothie: 5.6g Protein; 40.7g Carbohydrate; 3.1g Fat; and 10.9g Dietary Fibre.

| Essential Vitamins | | | | | | | | | | | | | Essential Minerals (and Iron) | | | | | |
A	B1	B2	B3	B5	B6	B7	B9	B12	C	D	E	K	CALC	MAG	PHOS	POT	SOD	IRON

Banana Smoothie

The Banana Smoothie packs a big potassium punch.

What you need:
1 banana
1 tbsp porridge oats
150ml milk (long life milk can be used - dairy, soy or any other
  alternatives available to you).
1 tsp honey
1 tsp vanilla extract

How to make it: Put the ingredients in the blender and mix until it is smooth and free from unwanted lumps.
There are approximately 205 calories in the Banana Smoothie: 8.3g Protein; 38.4g Carbohydrate; 1.9g Fat; and 3.3g Dietary Fibre.

Essential Vitamins													Essential Minerals (and Iron)					
A	B1	B2	B3	B5	B6	B7	B9	B12	C	D	E	K	CALC	MAG	PHOS	POT	SOD	IRON
		X		X	X	X		X					X	X		X		X

Green Smoothie

Try this tasty breakfast smoothie to start your day.

What you need:
160g ripe strawberries
160g baby spinach
1 small avocado, halved and the flesh scooped out
2 small oranges, juiced, plus ½ tsp finely grated zest
150ml pot bio yogurt – this is the tricky ingredient.

How to make it: Put the ingredients in the blender and mix until it is smooth and free from unwanted lumps.

There are approximately 384 calories in the Green Smoothie: 19g Protein; 37.1g Carbohydrate; 16.2g Fat; and 8.6g Dietary Fibre.

Essential Vitamins													Essential Minerals (and Iron)					
A	B1	B2	B3	B5	B6	B7	B9	B12	C	D	E	K	CALC	MAG	PHOS	POT	SOD	IRON

There are some bio-yogurt/bio-drinks that do not need to be refrigerated, and others that can be reconstituted with water. If you use one of these, please be careful with food safety and remember that heat can reduced the bioactivity of microorganisms contained in the product. Alternatively, this can be made at a time when you have access to refrigerated yoghurt (unsweetened or Greek yoghurt is preferable) and the smoothie carried in a thermal drink container.

Another Green smoothie

Green smoothies are very healthy, so here is another version for you to try. Add protein powder if you would like to increase the protein content of this smoothie.

What you need:
200ml soy milk
60g spinach
1 banana (small, peeled, sliced, frozen)
1 mango
1/2 avocado (small, sliced)

How to make it: Put the ingredients in the blender and mix until it is smooth and free from unwanted lumps.

There are approximately 501 calories in Another Green Smoothie (without protein powder): 34.2g Protein; 53.5g Carbohydrate; 15.5g Fat; and 8.4g Dietary Fibre.

Essential Vitamins													Essential Minerals (and Iron)					
A	B1	B2	B3	B5	B6	B7	B9	B12	C	D	E	K	CALC	MAG	PHOS	POT	SOD	IRON
▓	▓	▓	▓	▓	▓	▓	▓	▓	▓		▓		▓	▓		▓	▓	▓

If you choose milk that is fortified with vitamin D, you can increase your vitamin D intake with this smoothie. If you live in an area where you are outside in sunlight, you may receive adequate sunlight on your skin to meet your body's vitamin D requirements. However, if you live in remote areas where there are long winters and limited sunlight fortified milk products may help you with your body's vitamin D requirements.

Fruit Smoothie

This is a simple smoothie that is easy to make in the morning if you are in a hurry. It would be a great in an insulated drink container as an on-the-go breakfast for those early starts!

What you need:
10 strawberries (approx 175g)
1 medium banana
150ml orange juice

How to make it: Put the ingredients in the blender and mix until it is smooth and free from unwanted lumps.

Tip: Add protein powder to make this a high protein snack.

There are approximately 332 calories in the Fruit Smoothie: 15g Protein; 46.7g Carbohydrate; 7.5g Fat; and 5.2g Dietary Fibre.

Essential Vitamins													Essential Minerals (and Iron)					
A	B1	B2	B3	B5	B6	B 7	B9	B12	C	D	E	K	CALC	MAG	PHOS	POT	SOD	IRON

Tropical smoothie

This is another smoothie that would be a great in an insulated drink container as an on-the-go breakfast or morning snack! If you have access to a freezer, it can be made the night before and frozen overnight. Depending on the temperature in which you work, you will have a thick smoothie to drink sometime between leaving home and morning tea time!

What you need:
3 peeled kiwi fruit
1 mango, peeled, stoned and chopped
200ml pineapple juice
1 banana, sliced

How to make it:
Put the ingredients in the blender and mix until it is smooth and free from unwanted lumps.

Tip: Add spirulina to make this a more nutrient dense snack, or add protein powder to make this a high protein snack.

There are approximately 379 calories in the Tropical Smoothie: 6.8g Protein; 79g Carbohydrate; 1g Fat; and 13.6g Dietary Fibre.

| Essential Vitamins | | | | | | | | | | | | | Essential Minerals (and Iron) | | | | | |
A	B1	B2	B3	B5	B6	B7	B9	B12	C	D	E	K	CALC	MAG	PHOS	POT	SOD	IRON

CHAPTER SEVEN: SOUPS

Soups are a great way to add nutrients to your day, and all you need is a thermos or access to hot water for these satisfying soupy snacks. You can start with a soup base and then add nutrient dense foods based on what is available to you. Alternatively, use a packet soup as your base.

Where fresh ingredients are possible, they are the best option and adding fresh herbs (e.g. parsley) is another way to add nutrients. Where fresh foods are not available, this chapter offers some ideas to add nutrients to standard instant soup recipes.

Soup bases

Store bought instant soups

There are many varieties of low salt and/or low fat cup-of-soup type varieties available in stores. These can make a great soup base with premeasured sachets making them an easy snack for busy people. Then, you add your own foods to increase the taste and the nutritious value of the soup.

Make your own soup base

You can make you own soup base using stock cubes, miso paste, or any other flavour-base that you like. Add curry, and spices to create something that you love! Then, make a larger quantity of your chosen combination and store it in an air tight container. You can then scoop out 1-2 tablespoons of the mix and put it in your thermos or soup drink bottle.

Adding nutrients to soup bases

Following are some ideas for adding nutrients when you are in working remote areas.

Take pre-measured quantities of dehydrated vegetables in small containers or snap lock bags to work so that you can just add them to the soup base and hot water. Foods that can be dehydrated easily, and taste good in soups include: spring onions, corn, mushrooms, carrots, celery, and tomatoes. You are only limited by your imagination, and the capacity of the dehydrator.

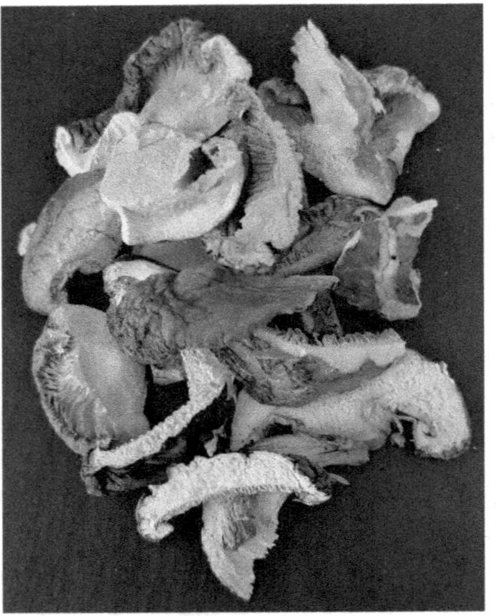

Store bought pre-dried or freeze-dried vegetables can be added and require less effort than dehydrating them yourself.

Preserved vegetables (e.g. mushrooms, tomatoes) can be added to soups. If you do not wish to preserve your own, store bought preserved (or pickled vegetables) can be used. If the vegetables are preserved in large jars of vegetables oil, you can measure smaller quantities into containers and take them to work with you to add to your soup.

Small cans of vegetables, such as corn, capsicum etc. are non-perishable and easy to transport. Add canned tuna or salmon for additional protein and omega-3 fatty acids.

Add grains such as barley, or lentils for added protein. Try adding rice noodles, such as rice vermicelli noodles which will cook in the hot water. Thenoodles can be stored in a container and then a portion added to the soup.

Chicken Noodle and Corn Soup

It is not quite like the one mum used to make but it will get you through a cold day.

What you need:
I sachet of instant chicken noodle soup
250ml boiling water
10g dehydrated corn
10g dehydrated carrot
5g dehydrated peas
5g dehydrated spring onion

How to make it:
Stir and leave for 2-3 minutes. The soup is ready when the corn and carrot is reconstituted and it is cool enough to drink.

There are approximately 68 calories in the Chicken Noodle and Corn Soup: 2g Protein; 11.5g Carbohydrate; 1.1g Fat; and 1.2g Dietary Fibre.

ESSENTIAL VITAMINS													ESSENTIAL MINERALS					
A	B1	B2	B3	B5	B6	B7	B9	B12	C	D	E	K	CALC	MAG	PHOS	POT	SOD	IRON

Hearty Vegetable Soup

Put some thought into the soup base because it is the heart of this hearty soup. Some brands have instant soups that start with an array of vegetables which give you something tasty to add to with your choice of available vegetables. Consider adding lentils to this soup for added protein.

What you need:
I sachet of instant hearty vegetable soup
250ml boiling water
20g dehydrated corn
20g dehydrated carrot
20g dehydrated mushroom
15g dehydrated peas
15g dehydrated spring onion

How to make it:
Stir and leave for 2-3 minutes. The soup is ready when the corn and carrot is reconstituted and it is cool enough to drink.

There are approximately 217 calories in the Vegetable Soup: 5.9g Protein; 31g Carbohydrate; 6.6g Fat; and 3.1g Dietary Fibre.

ESSENTIAL VITAMINS													ESSENTIAL MINERALS					
A	B1	B2	B3	B5	B6	B7	B9	B12	C	D	E	K	CALC	MAG	PHOS	POT	SOD	IRON

Chunky Minestrone-like Soup

This is not a traditional minestrone soup, but if you find a base with strong flavours it will get you through a cold afternoon. The soup pasta (it is a real thing) can be replaced with rice noodles, or barley.

What you need:
I sachet of instant Minestrone soup
250ml boiling water
20g dehydrated celery
20g dehydrated carrot
20g dried/dehydrated tomato
15g soup pasta

How to make it:
1) Put 50ml into a cup and add the soup pasta. Leave for 4 minutes or the length of time as per the instructions on the soup pasta packet (approx 4-6 minutes).
2) Add dehydrated vegetables and the sachet of instant soup and then add the other 200ml of boiling water.
3) The soup should be ready in about two minutes.

There are approximately 202 calories in the Chunky Minestrone Soup: 4.2g Protein; 36.8g Carbohydrate; 3g Fat; and 1.7g Dietary Fibre.

ESSENTIAL VITAMINS													ESSENTIAL MINERALS					
A	B1	B2	B3	B5	B6	B7	B9	B12	C	D	E	K	CALC	MAG	PHOS	POT	SOD	IRON

SECTION THREE: ABOUT THE NUTRIENTS

'Nothing tastes as good as healthy feels'

Anonymous

CHAPTER EIGHT: VITAMINS AND MINERALS – WHAT THEY DO AND WHERE THEY ARE FOUND

<u>About the essential vitamins</u>

The table below is a summary of the essential vitamins that an average male and female, aged 19 years or more, with good health require daily to maintain their good health. These are the nutrient requirements that have been used for the calculations in this book.

The following pages list the essential vitamin with a description of the role they play in maintaining good health. In addition, there is a list of good sources of the nutrient for people who work in remote and isolated areas.

Essential Vitamins	Recommended Daily Requirements		
	Age	RDI	AI
Vitamin A	Men (>19 years)	900mg	
(Retinoid and Carotene)	Women (>19 years)	700mg	
Vitamin B1	Men (>19 years)	1.2mg	
(Thiamin)	Women (>19 years)	1.1mg	
Vitamin B2	Men (>19 years)	1.3mg	
(Riboflavin)	Women (>19 years)	1.1mg	
Vitamin B3	Men (>19 years)	16mg	
(Niacin)	Women (>19 years)	14mg	
Vitamin B5	Men (>19 years)	6mg	
(Panthothenic Acid)	Women (>19 years)	4mg	
Vitamin B6	Men (19-50 years)	1.3mg	
	Men (>50 years)	1.7mg	
	Women (19-50 years)	1.3mg	
	Women (>50 years)	1.5mg	
Vitamin B7	Men (>19 years)		30mg
(Biotin)	Women (>19 years)		25mg
Vitamin B9	Men (>19 years)	400mg	
(Folate)	Women (>19 years)	400mg	
Vitamin B12	Men (>19 years)	2.4mcg	
	Women (>19 years)	2.4mcg	
Vitamin C	Men (>19 years)	45mg	
	Women (>19 years)	45mg	
Vitamin D	Men (19-50 years)		5 mg
	Men (51-70 years)		10mg
	Men (>70 years)		15mg
	Women (19-50 years)		5 mg
	Women (51-70 years)		10mg
	Women (>70 years)		15mg
Vitamin E	Men (>19 years)		10mg
	Women (>19 years)		7mg
Vitamin K	Men (>19 years)		70mg
	Women (>19 years)		60mg

Vitamin A (Retinoid and Carotene)

Vitamin A is a fat-soluble vitamin. It is essential for vision, healthy skin, normal reproduction, and plays an important role in bone growth and the immune system (NHMRC and MOH, 2014; Sarris and Wardle, 2014).

The estimated amount of dietary Vitamin A required to maintain a well-nourished person of average body size is shown in this table (Commonwealth of Australia 2006).

Vitamin A		RDI
Men		
	>19 years	900 µg/day
Women		
	>19 years	700 µg/day

Good sources of Vitamin A (from 100g of food) include:
- Sweet potatoes (approximately 961µg)
- Carrots (approximately 852µg)
- Bluefin tuna (approximately 757µg)
- Romaine Lettuce (approximately 436µg)
- Chives (approximately 218µg)
- Spinach (approximately 469µg)
- Parsley (approximately 421µg)
- Garden Cress (approximately 346µg)
- Rock melon/cantaloupe (approximately 169µg)
- Sweet Red Bell Peppers (approximately 157µg).

When you live and work in a remote area, some of the good sources can be difficult to access; however, there are non-perishable foods rich in Vitamin A: canned salmon, canned oysters, tomato paste, sun-dried tomatoes, and Spirulina (dried seaweed).

Vitamin B1 (Thiamin)

Thiamin is a water-soluble vitamin that occurs in most plant and animal foods. It plays an essential role in the supply of energy and nerve function (NHMRC and MOH, 9 April 2014a). It is also important for healthy skin, hair, muscles, and brain function. Thiamin is found predominantly in cereal foods. In Australia, there is mandatory thiamin enrichment of baking flour (NHMRC and MOH, 9 April 2014a).

The estimated amount of dietary vitamin B1 required to maintain a well-nourished person of average body size is shown in this table (Commonwealth of Australia 2006).

Vitamin B1	
	RDI
Men	
>19 years	1.2 mg/day
Women	
>19 years	1.1 mg/day

Good sources of Vitamin B1 (from 100g of food) are:
- Flax Seeds (approximately 1.6 mg)
- Lean Pork Chops (approximately 0.7mg)
- Salmon (approximately 0.3 mg)
- Green Peas (approximately 0.3 mg)
- Mussels (approximately 0.3 mg)
- Firm Tofu (approximately 0.2 mg)
- Brown Rice (approximately 0.2 mg)

When you live and work in a remote area, some of the good sources can be difficult to access; however, there are non-perishable foods rich in Vitamin B1: canned salmon, canned or dried peas, lentils, canned beans, and sunflower seeds.

Vitamin B2 (Riboflavin)

Vitamin B2, more commonly known as Riboflavin, is a water-soluble vitamin. Riboflavin helps to convert food into energy and is therefore, an essential vitamin for energy metabolism and a wide variety of cellular processes (NHMRC and MOH, 9 April 2014b). It is also needed for healthy skin and hair. The bioactive forms of riboflavin function as co-enzymes for key reactions in the catabolism of fuel molecules and in certain biosynthetic pathways (NHMRC and MOH, 9 April 2014b).

The estimated amount of dietary Vitamin B2 (Riboflavin) required for maintaining a well-nourished person of average body size is shown in this table (Commonwealth of Australia 2006).

Vitamin B2		
		RDI
Men		
	>19 years	1.3 mg/day
Women		
	>19 years	1.1 mg/day

Good sources of Vitamin B2 (from 100g of food) are:
- Almonds (approximately 1.1mg)
- Beef (approximately 0.9mg)
- Salmon (approximately 0.5mg)
- Mushrooms (approximately 0.5mg)
- Eggs (approximately 0.5mg)
- Fortified Tofu (approximately 0.4mg)

When you live and work in a remote area, some of the good sources can be difficult to access; however, there are non-perishable foods that contain Vitamin B2: almonds, canned salmon, UHT Milk, dehydrated mushrooms, beef jerky, quinoa, and lentils.

Vitamin B3 (Niacin)

Vitamin B3, or niacin, is a water-soluble vitamin that is well regulated by the body. It is required for processing fat in the body, lowering cholesterol levels, and regulating blood sugar levels. It helps convert food into energy and is essential for healthy skin, blood cells, brain, and the nervous system (NHMRC and MOH, 9 April 2014c). People who eat high amounts of refined foods are at risk of Vitamin B3 (Niacin) Deficiency.

The estimated amount of dietary vitamin B3 (Niacin) required for maintaining a well-nourished person of average body size is shown in this table (Commonwealth of Australia 2006).

Vitamin B3	
	RDI
Men	
>19-70 years	16 mg/day
Women	
>19-70 years	14 mg/day

Good sources of Vitamin B3 (from 100g of food) are:
- Tuna (Yellowfin) (approximately 22.1 mg)
- Peanuts (Roasted, unsalted) (approximately 14.4 mg)
- Lean Chicken Breast (approximately 9.5 mg)
- Lean Pork Chops (approximately 8 mg)
- Portabella Mushrooms (approximately 6.3 mg)
- Beef (approximately 5.6 mg)
- Brown Rice (approximately 2.6 mg)
- Avocados (approximately 1.7 mg)

When you live and work in a remote area, some of the good sources can be difficult to access; however, there are non-perishable foods that contain Vitamin B3: canned tuna, peanuts, peanut butter/paste, brown rice, and dehydrated mushrooms.

Vitamin B5 (Panthothenic Acid)

Vitamin B5, or Pantothenic Acid, is a water-soluble vitamin. It is an essential vitamin for cellular processes because it helps convert food into energy (NHMRC and MOH, 9 April 2014d). It also helps make lipids (fats), neurotransmitters, steroid hormones, and hemoglobin (NHMRC and MOH, 9 April 2014d).

The estimated amount of dietary Vitamin B5 required for maintaining a well-nourished person of average body size is shown in the table (Commonwealth of Australia 2006).

Vitamin B5 (Panthothenic Acid)	
	RDI
Men	
>19 years	6 mg/day
Women	
>19 years	4 mg/day

Good sources of Vitamin B5 (from 100g of food) are:
- Sunflower Seeds (approximately 7 mg)
- Shiitake Mushrooms (approximately 3.6 mg)
- Salmon (approximately 1.9 mg)
- Lean Chicken Breast (approximately 1.6 mg)
- Avocados (approximately 1.4 mg)
- Beef (approximately 1.3 mg)
- Lentils (approximately 0.6 mg)
- Sweet Potatoes (approximately 0.5 mg)

When you live and work in a remote area, some of the good sources can be difficult to access; however, there are non-perishable foods that contain Vitamin B5: shiitake mushrooms (can be dehydrated and added to soups), lentils can be added to soups, canned salmon, sunflower seeds, UHT milk, and sweet potatoes (dehydrated as chips or cooked into savoury snacks).

Vitamin B6

Vitamin B6 is a water-soluble vitamin. It performs a wide variety of functions in the body and is a co-enzyme in several reactions (NHMRC and MOH, 31 January 2018). Vitamin B6 also plays a role in cognitive development, hemoglobin formation and maintaining normal levels of amino acids in the blood, and immune function. Vitamin B6 is also added to many foods, and in many western countries dietary Vitamin B6 is in fortified cereals, bread and some flours.

The estimated amount of dietary vitamin B6 required for maintaining a well-nourished person of average body size is shown in this table (Commonwealth of Australia 2006).

Vitamin B6		RDI
Men		
	19-50 years	1.3 mg/day
	>51 years	1.7 mg/day
Women		
	19-50 years	1.3 mg/day
	>51 years	1.5 mg/day

Good sources of Vitamin A (from 100g of food) are:
- Pistachios (approximately 1.7mg)
- Salmon (approximately 0.9mg)
- Lean Chicken Breast (approximately 0.9mg)
- Lean Pork Chops (approximately 0.5mg)
- Beef (approximately 0.5mg)
- Bananas (approximately 0.4mg)
- Avocados (approximately 0.3mg)

When you live and work in a remote area, some of the good sources can be difficult to access; however, there are non-perishable foods that contain vitamin B6: canned salmon, sweet potatoes (dehydrated), pistachios, and bananas (dehydrated).

Vitamin B7 (Biotin)

Vitamin B7, or Biotin, is a water-soluble vitamin. It helps to convert food into energy, and is needed for healthy bones and hair. Biotin is less bio-available in cereals making it important for people with a vegetarian or vegan diet to ensure there is adequate dietary intake (Mock 1996). There is limited information about the biotin content of foods.

The estimated amount of dietary Biotin required for maintaining a well-nourished person of average body size is shown in this table (Commonwealth of Australia 2006).

Vitamin B7	
	AI
Men	
>19 years	30 μg /day
Women	
>19 years	25 μg /day

Good sources of Vitamin B7 (from 100g of food) are:
- Sunflower seeds (approximately 252 μg)
- Walnuts (approximately 87 μg)
- Pecans (approximately 65 μg)
- Rice bran (approximately 60 μg)
- Green peas (raw or dried) (approximately 34 μg)
- Barley (approximately 31 μg)
- Lentils (approximately 23 μg)
- Mushroom (approximately 16 μg)
- Banana (approximately 5.5 μg)

When you live and work in a remote area, some of the good sources can be difficult to access; however, the foods in the above list contains are non-perishable foods, or foods that can be dehydrated.

Vitamin B9 (Folate)

Vitamin B9, commonly known as folate or folic acid, is a water-soluble vitamin essential for body functions such as DNA synthesis and repair, cell division, and cell growth (especially new cell creation). If taken early in a pregnancy it can help to reduce brain and spinal birth defects (NHMRC and MOH, 9 April 2014e). Some countries (e.g. Australia, New Zealand) have started to fortify orange juice with Vitamin B9, increasing the amount of folate added to many diets.

The estimated amount of dietary vitamin B9 (Folate) required for maintaining a well-nourished person of average body size is shown in this table (Commonwealth of Australia 2006).

Vitamin B9 (Folate)	
	RDI
Men	
>19 years	400 mg/day
Women	
>19 years	400 mg/day

Good sources of Vitamin B9 (from 100g of food) are:
- Edamame (Green Soybeans) (approximately 311 mg)
- Lentils (approximately 181 mg)
- Avocados (approximately 81 mg)
- Mangos (approximately 43 mg)
- Lettuce (approximately 136 mg)
- Sweet Corn (approximately 42 mg)
- Oranges (approximately 30 mg)

When you live and work in a remote area, some of the good sources can be difficult to access; however, there are non-perishable foods that contain Vitamin B9: corn (dehydrated, canned), oranges (whole fruit), mango (dehydrated), edamame and lentils.

Vitamin B12

Vitamin B12 is a water-soluble vitamin that helps with red blood cell formation, neurological function, and DNA synthesis (Institute of Medicine, 1998). It assists in making new cells, breaking down fatty and amino acids, and protects nerve cells as well as aiding normal cell growth. Vitamin B12 is generally not found in plant foods, but fortified breakfast cereals are a readily available source of Vitamin B12 for vegan and vegetarian diets (Institute of Medicine 1998, Subar et al, 1998).

The estimated amount of dietary vitamin B12 required for maintaining a well-nourished person of average body size is shown in this table (Commonwealth of Australia 2006).

Vitamin B12	
	RDI
Men	
>19 years	2.4 µg/day
Women	
>19 years	2.4 µg/day

Good sources of Vitamin B12 (from 100g of food) are:
- Fortified Nutritional yeast (approximately 116.6 µg)
- Liver (approximately 85.7 µg)
- Fortified Cereals (approximately 21 µg)
- Mackerel (approximately 19 µg
- Crab (approximately 11.5 µg)
- Sardines (approximately 9 µg)
- Beef (approximately 5.9 µg)
- Eggs (approximately 1.1 µg)

When you live and work in a remote area, some of the good sources can be difficult to access; however, there are non-perishable foods that are Vitamin B12 fortified.

Vitamin C

Vitamin C is a water-soluble vitamin that is required for the biosynthesis of collagen, certain neurotransmitters; and protein metabolism (Schellhorn 2007; Carr and Frei 1999). It is an important physiological antioxidant, and also plays an important role in immune function and improves the absorption of iron (Gershoff 1993).

The estimated amount of dietary Vitamin C required for maintaining a well-nourished person of average body size is shown in this table (Commonwealth of Australia 2006).

Vitamin C	
	RDI
Men	
>19 years	45 mg/day
Women	
>19 years	45 mg/day

Good sources of Vitamin C (from 100g of food) are:
- Bell Peppers/Capsicum (approximately 128 mg)
- Kiwifruit (approximately 93 mg)
- Strawberries (approximately 59 mg)
- Oranges (approximately 53 mg)
- Kale (approximately 41mg)
- Tomato (approximately 23 mg)

When you live and work in a remote area, some of the good sources can be difficult to access; however, there are non-perishable foods that contain vitamin C: oranges (whole fruit) and dehydrated or freeze dried strawberries can be added to smoothies or trail mixes.

Vitamin D

Vitamin D is an oil soluble vitamin. It is helps to maintain normal blood levels of calcium and phosphorus which strengthen bones, and in the formation of teeth and bones. Vitamin D also plays a role in the immune system, healthy skin and maintaining muscle strength (NHMRC and MOH, 9 April 2014f). Ultraviolet (UV) light from the sun is necessary for the production of vitamin D in the skin and is the best natural source of Vitamin D (Fuller and Casparian, 2001).

The estimated amount of dietary Vitamin D required for maintaining a well-nourished person of average body size is shown in this table (Commonwealth of Australia 2006).

Vitamin D	
	AI
Men	
19-50 years	5 mg/day
51-70 years	10 mg/day
>70 years	15 mg/day
Women	
19-50 years	5 mg/day
51-70 years	10 mg/day
>70 years	15 mg/day

Good sources of Vitamin D (from 100g of food) are:
- Salmon (approximately 16.7 mg)
- Fortified Breakfast Cereal (approximately 8.3 mg)
- Fortified Milk / Yogurt (approximately 1.3 mg)
- Fortified Soy Milk (approximately 1.2 mg)
- Fortified Orange Juice (approximately 1 mg)

When you live and work in a remote area, some of the good sources can be difficult to access; however, there are non-perishable foods that contain Vitamin D: canned salmon, fortified UHT milk and soy products, and fortified orange juice.

Vitamin E

Vitamin E is a fat-soluble vitamin. It helps to prevent oxidative stress on the body. Adequate amounts of vitamin E can help protect against heart disease, cancer, and age-related eye damage (macular degeneration) (NHMRC and MOH, 9 April 2014g). The main source of Vitamin E is fats and oils.

The estimated amount of dietary Vitamin E required for maintaining a well-nourished person of average body size is shown in this table (Commonwealth of Australia 2006).

Vitamin E		
		AI
Men		
	>19 years	10 mg/day
Women		
	>19 years	7 mg/day

Good sources of Vitamin E (from 100g of food) are:
- Sunflower Seeds (approximately 26.1 mg)
- Almonds (approximately 25.6 mg)
- Olive Oil (approximately 14.4mg)
- Avocados (approximately 2.1 mg)
- Trout (approximately 2.8 mg)
- Prawn/shrimp (approximately 2.2mg)
- Kiwifruit (approximately 1.5 mg)

When you live and work in a remote area, some of the good sources can be difficult to access; however, there are non-perishable foods that contain Vitamin E: sunflower seeds, almonds, kiwifruit (whole fruit does not need refrigeration), and olive oil used for cooking and as a dressing on foods (it is available in 20ml plastic bottles that are great when travelling).

Vitamin K

Vitamin K is the family name for a series of essential fat-soluble compounds. Vitamin K is an essential vitamin required for protein modification and blood clotting. In fact, Vitamin K is best-known for its role in the maintenance of normal blood coagulation (NHMRC and MOH, 9 April 2014h).

The estimated amount of dietary Vitamin K required for maintaining a well-nourished person of average body size is shown in this table (Commonwealth of Australia 2006).

Vitamin K		
		AI
Men		
	>19 years	70 mg/day
Women		
	>19 years	60 mg/day

Good sources of Vitamin K (from 100g of food) are:
- Kale (approximately 817 mg)
- Lettuce (approximately 102 mg)
- Pickled Cucumber (approximately 77 mg)
- Asparagus (approximately 51 mg)
- Green (Snap) Beans (approximately 48 mg)
- Kiwifruit (approximately 40 mg)

When you live and work in a remote area, some of the good sources can be difficult to access; however, there are non-perishable foods that contain Vitamin K: kiwifruit (whole fruit doesn't need refrigeration), pre-packed or home-made pickled cucumber, sundried tomatoes, spring onions can be dehydrated and added to soups, ground cloves, dried sage, parsley, chilli peppers, bell peppers/capsicum (canned, preserved or dehydrated), and pine nuts.

About the essential Minerals

The table provides a summary of the essential minerals for an average male and female, aged 19 years or more. The trace mineral 'iron' has also been included in this section. These are the nutrient requirements used for the calculations in this book.

Minerals	Recommended Daily Requirements		
	AGE	RDI	AI
Essential Minerals			
Calcium	Men (19-70 years)		1000mg
	Men (>70 years)		1300mg
	Women (19-70 years)		1000mg
	Women (>70 years)		1300mg
Magnesium	Men (19-30 years)		400mg
	Men (>30 years)		420 mg
	Women (19-30 years)		310 mg
	Women (>30 years)		320 mg
Phosphorus	Men (>19 years)	1000 mg/day	
	Women (>19 years)	1000 mg/day	
Potassium	Men (>19 years)		3800mg
	Women (>19 years)		2800mg
Sodium	Men (>19 years)		460-920mg
	Women (>19 years)		460-920mg
Trace Minerals			
Iron	Men(>19 years)		8mg
	Women (19-50 years)		18mg
	Women (>50 years)		8mg

Individual requirements will differ. A calculator such as this one (https://www.nrv.gov.au/nutrients-energy-calc) can help with more personalised information.

Calcium

Calcium is required for the normal development and maintenance of the skeleton as well as for the proper functioning of neuromuscular and cardiac function. Calcium builds and protects bones and teeth, it helps with muscle contractions and relaxation, blood clotting, and the transmission of nerve impulses (NHMRC and MOH, 9 April 2014i). Also, calcium has a role in hormone and enzyme activity and helps with maintaining a healthy blood pressure.

The estimated amount of dietary Calcium required for maintaining a well-nourished person of average body size is shown in this table (Commonwealth of Australia 2006).

Calcium		
		AI
Men		
	19-70 years	1000 mg/day
	>70 years	1300 mg/day
Women		
	19-70 years	1000 mg/day
	>70 years	1300 mg/day

Good sources of calcium (from 100g of food) for people in remote areas include:

- Parmesan cheese (approximately 1184 mg)
- Firm Tofu (approximately 683 mg)
- Low-Fat Yogurt (approximately 199 mg)
- Skim Milk (approximately 122 mg)

When you live and work in a remote area, some of the good sources can be difficult to access; however, there are non-perishable foods that contain calcium: UHT milk, canned sardines, sesame seeds, chia seeds, canned salmon (with bones), almonds, edamame, and dried figs.

Magnesium

Magnesium is an essential mineral required by the body for maintaining normal muscle and nerve function as well as maintaining the immune system, good heart health and strong bones. Magnesium works with calcium in muscle contraction, blood clotting, and regulation of blood pressure. The kidneys play a central role in magnesium homeostasis (Quarme and Disks 1986). Protein may influence magnesium absorption.

The estimated amount of dietary Magnesium required for maintaining a well-nourished person of average body size is shown in this table (Commonwealth of Australia 2006).

Magnesium	AI
Men	
19-30 years	400mg/day
>31 years	420mg/day
Women	
19-30 years	310mg/day
>31 years	320mg/day

Good sources of magnesium (from 100g of food) include:
- Pumpkin Seeds (approximately 550 mg)
- Almonds (approximately 270 mg)
- Dark Chocolate (85% Cocoa) (approximately 228 mg)
- Tuna (approximately 64 mg)
- Brown Rice (approximately 44 mg)
- Avocados (approximately 29 mg)
- Bananas (approximately 27 mg)
- Non-Fat Yogurt (approximately 19 mg)

When you live and work in a remote area, some of the good sources can be difficult to access; however, there are non-perishable foods in the list: canned tuna, pumpkin seeds, and almonds.

Phosphorus

Phosphorus is the second most abundant inorganic element in the body. Phosphorus is an essential nutrient required for cell functioning, regulation of calcium, strong bones and teeth, and for making ATP (adenosine triphosphate) a molecule which provides energy to our cells. Phosphorus is so widespread in the food supply that dietary phosphorus deficiency is extremely rare, the exception being long-term, severe food restriction (NHMRC and MOH, 9 April 2014j).

The estimated amount of dietary Phosphorus required to maintain a well-nourished person of average body size is shown in this table (Commonwealth of Australia 2006).

Phosphorus		
		RDI
Men		
	>19 years	1000 mg/day
Women		
	>19 years	1000 mg/day

Good sources of Phosphorus (from 100g of food) are:
- Pumpkin Seeds (approximately 1233mg)
- Tuna (Yellowfin) (approximately 333mg)
- Lean Pork Chops (approximately 303mg)
- Lean Chicken Breast (approximately 241mg)
- Beef (approximately 197mg)
- Lentils (approximately 180mg)
- Quinoa (approximately 152mg)

When you live and work in a remote area, some of the good sources can be difficult to access; however, there are non-perishable foods that contain phosphorus: canned tuna (Yellowfin), UHT Milk, pumpkin seeds, lentils and quinoa.

Potassium

Potassium helps to maintain the fluid and electrolyte balance in the body. It helps to maintain a regular heartbeat, and is needed for muscle contractions. A diet rich in potassium may improve blood pressure and benefit bones (NHMRC and MOH, 9 April 2014k).

The estimated amount of dietary potassium required to maintain a well-nourished person of average body size is shown in this table (Commonwealth of Australia 2006).

Potassium	
	AI
Men	
>19 years	3,800mg/day
Women	
>19 years	2,800mg/day

Good sources of Potassium (from 100g of food) are:
- Salmon (approximately 628 mg
- Large White Beans (approximately 561mg)
- Potatoes (approximately 535 mg)
- Avocados (approximately 485 mg)
- Bananas (approximately 358 mg)
- White Button Mushrooms (approximately 356 mg)
- Tomato (approximately 218 mg)
- Milk (approximately 150 mg)

When you live and work in a remote area, some of the good sources can be difficult to access; however, there are non-perishable foods that contain potassium: brazil nuts, canned tuna (Yellowfin), canned salmon, UHT milk, white button mushrooms (dehydrated), bananas, sundried tomatoes, sweet potatoes and beetroots (dehydrated into chips), edamame and dried apricots.

Sodium

Sodium is everywhere in the food supply and is essential in human physiology. However, excess sodium intakes have been associated with increased chronic disease risk, and high blood pressure (NHMRC 2013). Sodium balance is maintained through a range of physiological and hormonal systems. Sodium is largely consumed as sodium chloride, or 'salt'. Sodium may also be found in food additives such as sodium phosphate, sodium bicarbonate and sodium benzoate. Fast food, dairy products, cereals, pasta, biscuits, cake, and meat products contribute significantly to sodium intake (MoH 2003, NZFSA 2005).

The estimated amount of Sodium required to maintain a well-nourished person of average size is shown in this table (Commonwealth of Australia

Sodium	
	AI*
Men	460-920 mg/day
Women	460-920 mg/day

2006). The AI for sodium is the amount required to ensure that basic requirements are met and to allow for adequate intake of other nutrients.

Good sources of sodium (from 100g of food) are:
- Table Salt (approximately 38,758 mg)
- Sunflower Seeds (approximately 6008mg)
- Soy Sauce (approximately 5493 mg)
- Canned Anchovies (approximately 3668 mg)
- Chili Powder (approximately 2867 mg)

When you live and work in a remote area, the healthiest source of sodium is sea salt, with iodised table salt being a good source of both iodine and sodium.

Iron

Iron is an essential mineral which helps hemoglobin in red blood cells and myoglobin in muscle cells to transport oxygen throughout the body. Women of childbearing age have higher dietary requirements for iron, therefore, in some countries foods are fortified to increase the amount of iron consumed in the average diet (NHMRC and MOH, 9 April 2014l).

The estimated amount of dietary Iron required for maintaining a well-nourished person of average body size is shown in this table (Commonwealth of Australia 2006).

Iron	
	AI
Men	
>19-70 years	8 mg/day
Women	
19-50 years	18 mg/day
>51 years	8 mg/day

Good sources of Iron (from 100g of food) are:
- Fortified Cereals (approximately 67.7mg)
- Baking Chocolate (approximately 17.4 mg)
- Dried Apricots (approximately 6.3 mg)
- Beef (approximately 5.5 mg)
- Quinoa (approximately 1.5 mg)
- Pumpkin Seeds (approximately 8.8mg)

When you live and work in a remote area, some of the good sources can be difficult to access; however, there are non-perishable foods that contain iron: dried apricots, quinoa, pumpkin seeds, dark chocolate, and fortified cereals which can be used in baking as well as for breakfast!

SECTION FOUR: MY RESOURCES, MY SNACKS

Knowledge is a tool, and like all tools, its impact is in the hands of the user.

Dan Brown

CHAPTER NINE: TEMPLATES AND PLANNERS

'Motivation Is What Gets You Started. Habit Is What Keeps You Going'
Jim Rohn

Trail mix templates

When building your own Trail Mix, you can use this template to mark the boxes for the nutrients contained in each food. For example, if you choose Almonds, you would tick the boxes as per the example below:

Ingredient (100g)	ESSENTIAL VITAMINS													ESSENTIAL MINERALS					
	A	B1	B2	B3	B5	B6	B7	B9	B12	C	D	E	K	CALC	MAG	PHOS	POT	SOD	IRON
Almond	✓	✓	✓	✓	✓	✓		✓				✓		✓	✓	✓	✓	✓	✓

This will help you to see that the foods you are choosing contain most of the nutrients. Please be aware that it may be difficult to get foods with vitamin B7, B12 and D in your Trail Mix, but there are other ways to include these nutrients in other meals to balance your nutrient intake across the day.

To calculate the quantities for your trail mix, use the 'My Personal Trail Mix Template', and calculate the total for each nutrient. Next, find the RDI/AI for the age group that includes your current age in the table in Chapter Eight. Then divide the total for each nutrient in your Trail Mix (marked with the letter 'A' in the template) by the daily RDI/AI for a person of your gender and age. For example, if I was a 35 year old woman, the RDI for vitamin B9 is 400mg. So I would divide the amount in A by 400 and multiply by 100 to get the percentage of the daily RDI.

MY PERSONAL TRAIL MIX 'TEMPLATE'																								
Foods (100g)	MACRO					ESSENTIAL VITAMINS													ESSENTIAL MINERALS (and Iron)					
	CAL	PROT	CARB	FAT	FIBRE	A	B1	B2	B3	B5	B6	B7	B9	B12	C	D	E	K	CALC	MAGN	PHOS	POT	SOD*	IRON
TOTAL¹																								
100g portion²	A	A	A	A	A	A	A	A	A	A	A	A	A	A	A	A	A	A	A	A	A	A	A	A

% of RDI/AI³																								

¹The total is assumed to be for 500g of Trail Mix
²Divide the total by 5 to get the nutrient amounts for a 100g portion of Trail Mix
³This is the portion for you, use the summary in Chapter Eight to work out the quantity for you

Email the author if you would like a fillable copy of these templates emailed directly to you:
helpingremotemanagers@gmail.com

An overview of the nutrients contained in individual Trail Mix ingredients

The next table has the quantities for the foods in the suggested Trail Mixes to help you to estimate the percentage of the RDI/AI for each nutrients you added to included in your Trail Mix. Not everyone will want to do this, but if you like this type of thing – have fun with it!

	MACRO				ESSENTIAL VITAMINS													ESSENTIAL MINERALS & IRON					
100g food (unless otherwise stated)	PROTEIN	CARBOHYDRATE	FAT	FIBRE	A (RETINOL)	B1 (THIAMIN)	B2 (RIBOFLAVIN)	B3 (NIACIN)	VITAMIN B5	VITAMIN B6	B7 (BIOTIN)	B9 (FOLATE)	VITAMIN B12	VITAMIN C	VITAMIN D	VITAMIN E	VITAMIN K	CALCIUM	MAGNESIUM	PHOSPHORUS	POTASSIUM	SODIUM	IRON
	g	g	g	g	ug	mg	mg	mg	mg	mg	ug	mg	ug	mg	ug	mg	mg	mg	mg	mg	mg	mg	mg
NUTS																							
Almond	21.2	21.7	49.4	12.2	1.0	0.2	1.0	3.4	0.5	0.1	45	50				26.2		264	268	484	705	1	3.7
Brazil nut	14.3	12.3	66.4	7.5		0.6		0.3	0.2	0.1		22		0.7		5.7		160	376	725	659	3	2.4
Cashew	18.2	32.7	43.8	3.3		0.4	0.1	1.1	0.9	0.4		25		0.5		0.9	34.1	37	292	593	660	12	6.7
Hazelnuts	15	16.7	60.7	9.7	20	0.6	0.1	1.8	0.9	0.6		113		6.3		15	14.2	114	163	290	680		4.7
Macadamia	7.9	14.2	75.8	8.6		1.2	0.2	2.5	0.8	0.3		11.0		1.2		0.5		85	130	188	368	5.0	3.7
Peanut	23.7	21.5	49.7	8.0		0.4	0.1	13.5	1.4	0.3	50	145				6.9		5	176	358	658	6	2.3
Pistachios	21.3	27.7	46	10.3	262	0.8	0.2	1.4	0.5	1.3		50		2.3		1.9	13.2	110	120	485	1042	10	4.2
Walnuts	15.2	13.7	65.2	6.7	20	0.3	0.2	1.1	0.6	0.5	2.8	98		1.3		0.7	2.7	98	158	346	441	2.0	2.9
FRUIT																							
Apricot (dried)	3.4	62.6	0.5	7.3	3604		0.1	2.6		0.1		10		1		4.3	3.1	55	32	71	1162	10	2.7
Apple (dried)	0.9	65.9	0.3	8.7			0.2	0.9	0.2	0.1				3.9		0.5	3	14	16	38	450	87	1.4
Banana chips	2.3	58.4	33.6	7.7	83	0.1		0.7	0.6	0.3	5.5	14		6.3		0.2	1.3	18	76	56	536	6.0	1.3
Blueberries (dried)	2.5	80	1.25	2.5	500			0.4	0.1			6		2		0.6	19.3	250	6	12	77	25	1.0
Cranberries (dried)	0.1	82.4	1.4	5.7				1.0	0.2					0.2		1.1	3.8	10	5.0	8.0	40	3.0	0.5
Dates (pitted)	1.8	75	0.2	6.7	149	0.1	0.1	1.6	0.8	0.2		15				2.7		64	54	62	696	1.0	0.9
Goji berries	11	21	1.0	8.0	9000	0.1	1.3							19.2				100			840	24	9.0
Mango (dried)	0.5	17	0.3	1.8	765	0.1	0.1	0.6	0.2	0.1		14		27.7		1.1	4.2	10	9.0	11.0	156	2.0	0.1
Pineapple (dried)	0.5	13.1	0.1	1.4	58	0.1		0.5	0.2	0.1		18		47.8		0.7		13	12	8	109	1.0	0.3
Raisins	3.1	79.2	0.5	3.7		0.1	0.1	0.8	0.1	0.2		5.0		2.3		0.1	3.5	50	32	101	749	11	1.9
Sultanas	2.4	74.2	0.2	8.2																	810	46	
Edamame	10.3	9.8	4.7	4.8		0.2	0.3	0.9	0.5	0.1		303		9.7		0.7	31.4	60	61	161	482	6.0	2.1
SEEDS & GRAINS																							
Flaxseeds	18.3	28.9	42.2	27.3		1.6	0.2	3.1	1.0	0.5		87		0.6		0.3	4.3	255	392	942	813	30	5.7
Pumpkin seeds	18.5	53.7	19.4		62		0.1	0.3	0.1			9.0		0.3				55	262	92	919	18	3.3
Sesame seeds (9g)	1.6	2.1	4.5	1.1	0.8	0.1		0.4		0.1		8.7						87.8	31.6	56.6	42.1	1.0	1.3
Sunflower seeds	20.8	20.0	57.5	8.6	50	1.5	0.4	8.3	1.1	1.3	5.7	227		1.4		33.2		78	325	660	645	9	5.2
Bran Cereal	9.4	80.4	2.2	17.6	2500	1.3	1.4	16.7	0.9	1.7		333	5.0		133	0.9	1.4	56	214	508	616	732	27
Puffed rice	7.0	87.8	0.9	1.4		0.4	0.3	3.5	0.3			154				0.1	0.1	9.0	30	118	116	5.0	2.9
Pretzels	10.3	79.2	2.6	3.0		0.5	0.3	5.1	0.3			186				0.4	2.1	18	29	113	136	1357	5.2
EXTRAS																							
Chili powder (8g)	0.9	4.1	1.3	2.6	2224		0.1	0.6		0.3		7.5		4.8		2.2	7.9	20.9	12.8	22.7	144	78.5	1.1
Cinnamon (8g)	0.3	6.2	0.1	4.1	22.9			0.1				0.5		0.3		0.2	2.4	77.7	4.7	5.0	33.4	0.8	0.6
Curry powder (6g)	0.8	3.6	0.9	2.1	61.6			0.2		0.1		9.6		0.7		1.4	6.2	29.9	15.9	21.8	96.4	3.2	1.8
Nutmeg (7g)	0.4	3.5	2.5	1.5	7.1			0.1				5.3		0.2				12.9	12.8	14.9	2.5	1.1	0.2
Onion Powder (7g)	0.7	5.4	0.1	0.4						0.1		11.2		1.0			0.3	24.5	8.2	22.9	63.7	3.6	0.2
Cacao Nibs	14.3	35.7	42.9	32.1		0.1	0.1	0.7	0.4	0.1			0.2				8.6	71.4	229	321	750		3.9
Chocolate (dark)	7.8	45.8	45.8	10.9	39		0.1	1.1	0.4					0.3			7.3	73	228	306	715	20	11.9
Coconut Flakes (15g)	1.0	4.0	10.0	2.0																			0.4
Choc Coffee beans	7.5	60	30	7.5			0.3	0.6	0.1			3.0				0.2	5.9	100	107	135	342	25	2.7

Email the author at :

helpingremotemanagers@gmail.com if you would like a copy of the 'An overview of the nutrients contained in individual Trail Mix ingredients' spreadsheet emailed to you.

Daily nutrients requirements by gender for two sample ages (30 years and 50 years)

Gender Age	Calories	MACRO NUTRIENTS				ESSENTIAL VITAMINS													ESSENTIAL MINERALS & IRON					
		PROTEIN	CARBOHYDRATE	FAT	FIBRE	A (RETINOL)	B1 (THIAMIN)	B2 (RIBOFLAVIN)	B3 (NIACIN)	VITAMIN B5	VITAMIN B6	B 7 (BIOTIN)	B9 (FOLATE)	VITAMIN B12	VITAMIN C	VITAMIN D	VITAMIN E	VITAMIN K	CALCIUM	MAGNESIUM	PHOSPHORUS	POTASSIUM	SODIUM	IRON
		g	g	g	g	RDI	RDI	RDI	RDI	RDI	RDI	AI	RDI	RDI	RDI	AI	AI	AI	AI	RDI	RDI	AI	AI	AI
Male																								
30 years	2500	750	1000	750	30	900	1.2	1.3	16	6	1.3	30	400	2.4	45	5	10	70	1000	400	1000	3800	460	8
50 years	2500	750	1000	750	30	900	1.2	1.3	16	6	1.7	30	400	2.4	45	10	10	70	1000	420	1000	3800	460	8
Female																								
30 years	2000	600	800	600	25	700	1.1	1.1	14	4	1.3	25	400	2.4	45	5	7	60	1000	310	1000	2800	460	18
50 years	2000	600	800	600	25	700	1.1	1.1	14	4	1.5	25	400	2.4	45	10	7	60	1000	320	1000	2800	460	8

Building a Trail Mix Template

Ingredient (100g)	ESSENTIAL VITAMINS													ESSENTIAL MINERALS					
	A	B1	B2	B3	B5	B6	B 7	B9	B12	C	D	E	K	CALC	MAG	PHOS	POT	SOD	IRON

Email the author if you would like a copy of the 'Building a Trail Mix Template' emailed to you at:
helpingremotemanagers@gmail.com

Daily planner

Food	MACRO				ESSENTIAL VITAMINS													ESSENTIAL MINERALS					Calories
	PROTEIN	CARBOHYDRATE	FAT	FIBRE	A (RETINOL)	B1 (THIAMIN)	B2 (RIBOFLAVIN)	B3 (NIACIN)	VITAMIN B5	VITAMIN B6	B 7 (BIOTIN)	B9 (FOLATE)	VITAMIN B12	VITAMIN C	VITAMIN D	VITAMIN E	VITAMIN K	CALCIUM	MAGNESIUM	PHOSPHORUS	POTASSIUM	SODIUM	
Breakfast																							
Snack																							
Lunch																							
Snack																							
Dinner																							
TOTAL																							

Email the author if you would like a copy of 'Daily Planner' template emailed to you at:
helpingremotemanagers@gmail.com

SNACK BETTER, FEEL BETTER

Five-day Planner

Food		MACRO				ESSENTIAL VITAMINS													ESSENTIAL MINERALS					
		PROTEIN	CARBOHYDRATE	FAT	FIBRE	A (RETINOL)	B1 (THIAMIN)	B2 (RIBOFLAVIN)	B3 (NIACIN)	VITAMIN B5	VITAMIN B6	B7 (BIOTIN)	B9 (FOLATE)	VITAMIN B12	VITAMIN C	VITAMIN D	VITAMIN E	VITAMIN K	CALCIUM	MAGNESIUM	PHOSPHORUS	POTASSIUM	SODIUM	IRON
DAY 1	Breakfast																							
	Snack																							
	Lunch																							
	Snack																							
	Dinner																							
CONSUMED																								
DAY 2	Breakfast																							
	Snack																							
	Lunch																							
	Snack																							
	Dinner																							
CONSUMED																								
DAY 3	Breakfast																							
	Snack																							
	Lunch																							
	Snack																							
	Dinner																							
CONSUMED																								
DAY 4	Breakfast																							
	Snack																							
	Lunch																							
	Snack																							
	Dinner																							
CONSUMED																								
DAY 5	Breakfast																							
	Snack																							
	Lunch																							
	Snack																							
	Dinner																							
CONSUMED																								
WEEK SUMMARY																								

Email the author if you would like a copy of the 'Five-Day Planner' template emailed to you at:

helpingremotemanagers@gmail.com

REFERENCES

Anderson, R.A., Polansky, M.M., Bryden, N.A., Patterson, K.Y., Veillon, C., and Glinsmann, W.H. (1983) Effects of chromium supplementation on urinary Cr excretion of human subjects and correlation of Cr excretion with selected clinical parameters. *J Nutrition*, 113: 276–281.

Aoba, T. (1997) The Effect of Fluoride on Apatite Structure and Growth, *Critical Reviews in Oral Biology and Medicine*, 8(2): 136-153.

Aoba, T. and Fejerskov, O. (2002) Dental Fluorosis: Chemistry and Biology. *Critical Reviews in Oral Biology and Medicine*, 13(2): 155-170.

Australian Bureau of Statistics (ABS). (1998) *National Nutrition Survey. Nutrient intakes and physical measurements, Australia, 1995.* Australian Bureau of Statistics: Canberra.

Carr, A.C. and Frei, B. (1999) Toward a new recommended dietary allowance for vitamin C based on antioxidant and health effects in humans. *Am J Clin Nutr*, 69: 1086-1107.

Commonwealth of Australia. (2006) *Nutrient Reference Values for Australia and New Zealand Including Recommended Dietary Intakes.* ISBN 1864962437 (Online) Available at: https://www.nrv.gov.au/nutrients (accessed 2 July 2020).

Davis, M.l., Seaborn, C.D., and Stoecker, B.J. (1995) Effects of over-the-counter drugs on 51chromium retention and urinary excretion in rats. *Nutr Res*, 15: 201–210.

Fejerskov, O., Larsen, M.J., Richards, A., and Baelum V. (1994) Dental Tissue Effects on Fluoride, *Advances in Dental Research*, 8(1): 15-31.

Gershoff, S.N. (1993) Vitamin C (ascorbic acid): new roles, new requirements? Nutr Rev, 51: 313-326.

Food and Agricultural Organization (FAO). (2004) World Health Organization and United Nations University Expert consultation. *Report on human energy requirements*. FAO: Rome.

Fuller, K. and Casparian, J. (2001) Vitamin D: balancing cutaneous and systemic considerations. *Southern Med J*, 94: 58-64.

Institute of Medicine. Food and Nutrition Board. (1998) Dietary Reference Intakes: Thiamin, Riboflavin, Niacin, Vitamin B6, Folate, Vitamin B12, Pantothenic Acid, Biotin, and Choline. National Academy Press: Washington, DC.

Jack, B., Ayson, M., Lewis, S., Irving, A., Agresta, B., Ko, H., and Stoklosa, A. (2016) *Health Effects of Water Fluoridation: Evidence Evaluation Report*, Report to the National Health and Medical Research Council, Canberra.

King, J.C., Keen, C.L. and Zinc, In: Shils, M.E., Olsen, J.A.S., Shike, M., and Ross, A.C. (eds.) (1999) *Modern Nutrition in Health and Disease 9thedition*. Williams & Wilkins: Baltimore, 223–239.

Li, Y. and Schellhorn, H.E. (2007) New developments and novel therapeutic perspectives for vitamin C. *J Nutr*, 137: 2171-2184.

Ministry of Health (MOH). (1999) *NZ food: NZ People. Key results of the 1997 National Nutrition Survey*. Ministry of Health: Wellington.

Ministry of Health (MOH) and the University of Auckland. (2003) *Nutrition and the Burden of Disease: New Zealand 1997-2011*, Ministry of Health: Wellington.

National Health and Medical Research Council (NHMRC) (2013), *Australian Dietary Guidelines*. National Health and Medical Research Council: Canberra.

National Health and Medical Research Council (NHMRC) and Ministry of Health (MOH). (22 September 2017). Nutrient Values for Australia and New Zealand, Available at: https://www.nrv.gov.au/introduction (accessed 1 July 2020)

National Health and Medical Research Council (NHMRC) and Ministry of Health (MOH) (14 April 2014), 'Vitamin A', Nutrient Reference Values for Australia and New Zealand. Available https://www.nrv.gov.au/nutrients/vitamin-a (accessed 1 July 2020)

National Health and Medical Research Council (NHMRC) and Ministry of Health (MOH) (9 April 2014a), 'Thiamin', Nutrient Reference Values for Australia and New Zealand. Available at: https://www.nrv.gov.au/nutrients/thiamin (accessed 1 July 2020)

National Health and Medical Research Council (NHMRC) and Ministry of Health (MOH) (9 April 2014b), 'Riboflavin', Nutrient Reference Values for Australia and New Zealand. Available at: https://www.nrv.gov.au/nutrients/riboflavin (accessed 1 July 2020)

National Health and Medical Research Council (NHMRC) and Ministry of Health (MOH) (9 April 2014c), 'Niacin', Nutrient Reference Values for Australia and New Zealand. Available at: https://www.nrv.gov.au/nutrients/niacin (accessed 1 July 2020)

National Health and Medical Research Council (NHMRC) and Ministry of Health (MOH) (9 April 2014d), 'Pantothenic Acid', Nutrient Reference Values for Australia and New Zealand. Available at: https://www.nrv.gov.au/nutrients/pantothenic-acid (accessed 1 July 2020)

National Health and Medical Research Council (NHMRC) and Ministry of Health (MOH) (31 January 2018), 'Vitamin B6', Nutrient Reference Values for Australia and New Zealand. Available at: https://www.nrv.gov.au/nutrients/vitamin-b6 (accessed 1 July 2020)

National Health and Medical Research Council (NHMRC) and Ministry of Health (MOH) (9 April 2014e), 'Folate', Nutrient Reference Values for Australia and New Zealand. Available at: https://www.nrv.gov.au/nutrients/folate (accessed 1 July 2020)

National Health and Medical Research Council (NHMRC) and Ministry of Health (MOH) (9 April 2014f), 'Vitamin D', Nutrient Reference Values for Australia and New Zealand. Available at: https://www.nrv.gov.au/nutrients/vitamin-d (accessed 1 July 2020)

National Health and Medical Research Council (NHMRC) and Ministry of Health (MOH) (9 April 2014g), 'Vitamin E', Nutrient

Reference Values for Australia and New Zealand. Available at: https://www.nrv.gov.au/nutrients/vitamin-e (accessed 1 July 2020)

National Health and Medical Research Council (NHMRC) and Ministry of Health (MOH) (9 April 2014h), 'Vitamin K', Nutrient Reference Values for Australia and New Zealand. Available at: https://www.nrv.gov.au/nutrients/vitamin-k (accessed 1 July 2020)

National Health and Medical Research Council (NHMRC) and Ministry of Health (MOH) (9 April 2014i), 'Calcium', Nutrient Reference Values for Australia and New Zealand. Available at: https://www.nrv.gov.au/nutrients/calcium (accessed 1 July 2020)

National Health and Medical Research Council (NHMRC) and Ministry of Health (MOH) (9 April 2014j), 'Phosphorus', Nutrient Reference Values for Australia and New Zealand. Available at: https://www.nrv.gov.au/nutrients/phosphorus (accessed 1 July 2020)

National Health and Medical Research Council (NHMRC) and Ministry of Health (MOH) (9 April 2014k), 'Potassium', Nutrient Reference Values for Australia and New Zealand. Available at: https://www.nrv.gov.au/nutrients/potassium (accessed 1 July 2020)

National Health and Medical Research Council (NHMRC) and Ministry of Health (MOH) (9 April 2014l), 'Iron', Nutrient Reference Values for Australia and New Zealand. Available at: https://www.nrv.gov.au/nutrients/iron (accessed 1 July 2020)

New Zealand Food Safety Authority. (2005) *2003/04 New Zealand Total Diet Survey: Agricultural Compound Residues, Selected Contaminants and Nutrients*. New Zealand Food Safety Authority: Wellington.

Offenbacher, E.G. (1994) Promotion of chromium absorption by ascorbic acid. *Trace Elem Elect,* 11: 178–181.

Olivares, M. and Uauy, R. (1996) Limits of metabolic tolerance to copper and biological basis for present recommendations and regulations. *Am J Clin Nutr,* 63: 846S–852S.

Pennington, J.A.T. and Jones, J.W. (1987) Molybdenum, nickel, co-balt, vanadium and strontium in total diets. *J Am Diet Assoc*, 87: 1644–1650.

Quarme, G.A. and Disks, J.H. (1986) The physiology of renal magnesium handling. *Renal Physiol*, 9: 257–269.

Sarris, J. and Wardle, J. (2014) Clinical Naturopathy 2e, An evidence-based guide to practice. Elsevier, Australia.

Simpson, J.L., Bailey, L.B., Pietrzik, K., Shane, B., and Holzgreve, W. (2010) Micronutrients and women of reproductive potential: required dietary intake and consequences of dietary deficiency or excess. Part I - Folate, Vitamin B12, Vitamin B6. *J Matern Fetal Neonatal Med*, 23: 1323-1343.

Subar, A.F., Krebs-Smith, S.M., Cook, A., and Kahle, L.L. (1998) Dietary sources of nutrients among US adults, 1989 to 1991. *J Am Diet Assoc*, 98: 537-547.

Teng, F., Bito, T., Takenaka, S., Yabuta, Y., and Watanabe, F. (2016) Yolk of the Century Egg (Pidan) Contains a Readily Digestible Form of Free Vitamin B_{12}. *J Nutr Sci Vitaminol* (Tokyo), 62(5): 366-371.

Tsongas, T.A., Meglen, R.R., Walravens, P.A., and Chappell, W.R. (1980) Molybdenum in the diet: an estimate of average daily intake in the United States. *American Journal of Clinical Nutrition*, 33: 1103–1107.

Tucker, K.L., Olson, B., Bakun, P., Dallal, G.E., Selhub, J., and Rosenberg, I.H. (2004) Breakfast cereal fortified with folic acid, vitamin B-6, and vitamin B-12 increases vitamin concentrations and reduces homocysteine concentrations: a randomized trial. *American Journal of Clinical Nutrition*, 79(5): 805-811.

Turnlund, J.R., Keyes, W.R., Peiffer, G.L., and Scott, K.C. (1998) Copper absorption, excretion and retention by young men consuming low dietary copper determined by using the stable isotope Cu. *Am J Clin Nutr*, 67: 1219–1125.

Welch, R.M. and Carey, E.E. (1975) Concentration of chromium, nickel and vanadium in plant materials. *J Agric Food Chem*, 23: 479–482.

ABOUT THE AUTHOR

Leigh-Ann Onnis

Leigh-ann Onnis has authored a range of publications about remote health workforce sustainability, mental health and wellbeing, and people management. Her passion for supporting people who live and work in geographical remote and isolated areas is the driving force for her writing.

BOOKS BY THIS AUTHOR

Hrm And Remote Health Workforce Sustainability: The Influence Of Localised Management Practices

This book examines on the influence of localised management practices on workforce sustainability. For geographically remote managers, the book offers evidence-based information for developing effective management practices drawn from three separate, yet related research studies. The book provides insight into the human resource management challenges for remote managers, and provides resources and practical management tools for managers to localise their management practices.